When
Working Out
Isn't
Working Out

When Working Out Isn't Working Out

...

A Mind/Body Guide to Conquering Unidentified Fitness Obstacles

MICHAEL GERRISH

ST. MARTIN'S GRIFFIN 🐾 NEW YORK

Design by Helene Berinsky

Library of Congress Cataloging-in-Publication Data

Gerrish, Michael.
    When working out isn't working out : a mind/body guide to conquering unidentified fitness obstacles / Michael Gerrish.
        p.   cm.
    Includes bibliographical references.
    ISBN 0-312-19959-7
    1. Physical fitness.   2. Health.   3. Mind and body.   I. Title.
RA776.G455   1999
613.7—dc21   98-50055
                                                            CIP

First St. Martin's Griffin Edition: May 1999

10 9 8 7 6 5 4 3 2

To my wife, Cheryl Richardson,
and to my parents,
Curt and Pat Gerrish

Contents

Acknowledgments

As I think about all of the time and hard work that went into completing this book, I'm grateful for having so many good friends who were eager to lend their support. What I fear, though, is that because there are so many folks who deserve to be thanked, there's someone I've failed to acknowledge (who's going to assume he or she has been snubbed). So if your name isn't mentioned here, and you think you deserve to be thanked, I hope you'll excuse the oversight and pardon my absent mind.

Without rambling on any further, thank you to the following people: the very nice folks who run Gold's Gym in Salisbury, Massachusetts, in particular Eric Lever and the owners, John and Joanne. Thanks for supporting my work in the gym and for always treating me well.

My thanks to the Framingham Giants, in particular to Ed, Jon, Joe, Howard, Pete, Greg, Kevin, Steve, Adrian, Liam, and José, for the chance to escape, every now and then, from the rigors of writing this book. In addition, I'd like to thank Sharon Day and Susan Wormwood Forsley, for their inspirational E-mails and for being such faithful fans.

My appreciation also goes to Greg and Christine Barnes. Thanks for your kindness and friendship and for always keeping the faith. Also to Brother Bob Russell, for encouraging my success. Thanks for seeing the spark in me and for pointing me down the right road.

Special thanks are also due to the following colleagues and friends: Howard E. Stone, Jr., M.D., for his integrity, skill, and compassion; Susan Duggan, for being there and lending a caring ear; the Springfield gang—Jon Berg, Jon Younger, Sue Forsley, and Mikey D.; Pat Rogers, for being so good to me and helping me find my way; Fred Kamlot, my first client/guinea pig, "pig-out partner," and long-time friend; Ed Shea, Imago relationship coach, for his gentle, insightful advice; Niravi Payne, for making me mad (and for making me cut the crap); Joan Oliver and Marilyn Abraham, for their feedback on early drafts; George Carlin, for inspiring the mood of my ramblings in Chapter 3; my new friend, Gary "Bat" Mack (the best "sports shrink" in the West); and the lighthearted lama, Surya Das, for his wisdom and playful wit.

Thanks are due, in addition, to Patty Portwine and Ginger Burr, for always being so thoughtful and for being such wonderful friends. Also, thanks to Norb Carey, Paul Rogers, Teresa Consentino, Mark and Elaine Amundsen, Peter Valaskatgis, Linda Novotny, Stephen Cluney, Aryn Ekstedt, Gay Schoene, Ania O'Connor, Halé Baycu-Schatz, my great virtual assistant, Stacy Brice, and my parents in-law, John (Papazita) and Ann (Mamazita) Richardson, all of whom played an important role in making this book come true.

Special thanks to my "sister" and very attractive friend, Max Dilley, whose whimsical mind and creative soul always keep me amused and intrigued. Your lighthearted side (and intense side) is always a joy to "endure."

My heartfelt thanks to Jonathan Berg, the best chiropractor I know, as well as one of the very best friends that a person could ever have. Thanks for your unwavering faith and incessant votes of confidence. Thanks also for the adjustments, both to my attitude and to my spine.

My sincerest thanks to my spunky, crackerjack agent, Ashley Carroll, whose charmingly warped sense of humor frequently boosted my wobbly morale. Also thanks to David Smith, for adding his timely advice and for being the kind of advocate every author hopes to have.

I'm also very appreciative of the efforts of Heather Jackson, whose foresight and publishing instincts opened the door for me and this book. In addition, thanks to my editor at St. Martin's, Becky Koh, whose responsiveness and belief in this book made the process of writing it fun. And also thanks to John Murphy, Elaine Bleakney, and John Karle, as well as to Mark Resnick and the entire St. Martin's staff. Thanks for all the behind-the-scenes work and for getting behind this book.

A big thanks to all of my clients, who have helped me to love what I do. Thanks to all, past and present, for helping me grow and learn.

To the brothers three, Tom, Paul, and Chris, for deciding to cut me some slack. Thanks for not getting on my case (as much) as you normally would.

I would like to express special gratitude to my parents, Curt and Pat Gerrish, whose work ethic, strength, and integrity have been a guidepost for much of my work. Thanks for being so stubbornly sure that I have what it takes to succeed.

And finally, thanks to my gem of a wife, the most caring person I know, who makes me wonder, continually, what she's doing with someone like me. If marriages *are* made in heaven (and God is arranging the pairs), I can't help but think that, somehow, I must have done something right. Thank you Cheryl, for everything, with more love than words can say.

◆ ◆ ◆

Introduction:
Life in the Fat Lane

The Upside of Down

From our trials, we discover our trails.
—Marvel Elizabeth Harrison and Terry Kellogg

I t's not hard for me to remember what it was like to be ten years old. The things I remember best, in fact, are things that I'd like to forget. Things like my fifth-grade gym class. The memories I have of what it was like are disturbingly unimpaired; from the ache I felt deep in my heart when I was the last one picked for a team, to the sting that I felt as wet towels were repeatedly snapped on my naked behind. Harassed for being heavy, and teased because I was shy, essentially I was an outcast, a casualty of my flaws, the classic case of an overweight kid belittled, rejected, and shamed.

The abuse, it seemed, was unending, but it didn't just come from my peers. It was also from my gym teacher. On his *good* days, his disposition could have been likened to Marquis de Sade. Whether poking my pudgy, protruding paunch, or lifting my shirt to expose it, he was always making me look like a fool in front of my classmates and friends. He once even taped an article from a magazine to my locker. The headline read something like, "Too Much TV Takes Toll on Tubby Tots." As you might guess, I didn't care much for his manner of making a point.

Of all the bad memories I have of this time, there's one that is bittersweet. It's of a particular incident that marked a critical point in my life. It prompted the start of my lifelong quest to be optimally healthy and fit.

I was standing outside of the middle school gym on an overcast autumn day. While awaiting the start of gym class, I anxiously pondered my fate. Fearing the worst that could happen, I prayed that we weren't going to *run*. Of course this was wishful praying. On this day, we'd do just that; in fact, we'd be timed for speed.

As I waited my turn to compete for the title of "slowest kid in the class," I imagined how things would be different for me if I wasn't in such sorry shape. "I wonder how it would feel," I mused, "to be proud of the way I look, to be leaner, faster, and stronger, to know that I'm physically fit."

My thoughts then began to drift deeper as I entered a dreamlike state. It was then that I saw myself running, swiftly, like the wind, every movement effortless, every motion controlled. I pictured myself moving purposely, like a panther pursuing its prey. I imagined my thigh muscles rippling as my legs moved me faster and faster.

Next, I guided my fantasy to a highly unlikely conclusion. "What would it be like," I wondered, "to run faster than everyone else, to be praised, admired, and accepted, treated at last with *respect*?"

My daydream was interrupted by the harsh blast of a whistle. "Michael!" my gym teacher bellowed. "Get over here, you're next! It's your turn *now*. Are you ready?"

I was ready, all right. Ready to throw up. Making an effort to gather my wits, I stumbled my way to the line. I swallowed hard and then braced myself, awaiting the signal to start. All I could feel at that moment was the hard, heavy thump of my heart.

The loud, shrill sound of the whistle sent a cold shiver up my spine. As if I'd been shot from a cannon, I exploded away from the line. My legs began to churn wildly as I moved like a frightened cat. With every stride, I ran faster, as if fueled by a powerful force, as if at that moment I'd just been possessed by some restless, maniacal ghost. I couldn't have moved any faster if I'd been running to save my life.

I finally crossed the line, stumbling, falling, and struggling to catch my breath. I noticed my gym teacher shaking his watch and holding it up to his ear. He sneered as he stood with his hands on his hips, appearing both puzzled and stunned. "There must be some kind of mistake," he said. "That was the best time yet. You ran faster than everyone! Nobody else was close!"

"How can this be?" I thought to myself, at the same time bursting with pride. With a big, silly grin, I glanced back at him, expecting a few words of praise. At the very least, I thought I might get a "way-to-go" pat on the ass. "Are you sure your watch isn't broken?" I asked. "Are you sure that I ran that fast?"

"Yeah, I'm sure," he snarled, with a frown. "Impressed with yourself, *fat boy*?"

"Fat boy"?! My gym teacher called me *fat boy*! As my classmates howled with laughter, my eyes welled up with tears.

"That's it! I've had it," I said to myself. "I'm going to show them all! I'll make them all respect me if it's the last thing I ever do!"

So at the ripe old age of ten, I made a commitment to get in shape. Forthwith, I went on a diet, read countless books about exercise, and continually badgered whoever I could for advice about how to work out. Over and over again, I returned to the confines of my basement, where an exercise bike and some rusty old weights were consistently put to good use. I refused to be swayed from my goal. I was desperate to make myself stronger and I didn't care what it would take.

As time passed, I was pleased to find that my efforts were not in vain. As a result, I was fueled with hope and more confident that I'd succeed. Each little bit of progress gave me incentive to push myself more. "Nothing will stop me now," I thought. "Soon I'll surprise them all! No matter what happens, from this point on, I won't be mistreated again!"

A year or so later, I had my chance to prove that my work had paid off. It came the first time that I ever stepped foot in the exercise room at my school. It was a place I had always done well to avoid—until this particular day.

As I entered the room, I surveyed the scene and was shocked by what I observed. It surprised me to see that the school's strongest jocks had all gathered to test their strength. They were trying to lift what appeared to be an impressive amount of weight. I viewed the proceedings intently, entranced as I watched them all fail. Then, in a moment of madness, I blurted, "Hey, can I give it a try?"

A resounding chorus of laughter promptly echoed throughout the room. "What, are you kidding?" someone said. "You'd be lucky to move it an inch!"

The crowd mostly smirked and snickered as they moved to clear me a space. I knew I could lift a lighter weight. I had many times before. But I wasn't so sure I could lift this much weight, especially with everyone watching.

I positioned my hands on the cold steel bar, like I saw someone do on TV. Then, after taking a long, deep breath, I hoisted it from the floor. By the time the weight reached my shoulders, a hush had come over the crowd. I steadied myself. Finally, struggling with all I had left, I extended my wobbly arms. I then stood transfixed, like a statue, with the barbell held high overhead. I held it up proudly, as long as I could, underscoring my glorious feat. Much like the tale of Charles Atlas (the world's "most perfectly built" ex-wimp), I was finally able to gain some respect by displaying my newfound strength. It may have been just a moment, but it was one I'd never forget. It was a shining example of what I could do if only I dared to try.

My reason for sharing this story is mainly to offer a message of hope—to help you to see that you *can* change your fate, that there's often an *upside to down*. The experience involving my gym coach could have left me scarred for life. But instead it helped to empower me and provided incentive to change. Instead of it making me lose all hope, it inspired me to set a new goal. Instead of it making me weaker, it actually gave me strength. It served as a perfect example of how, sometimes, blessings come in disguise.

What if your setbacks were also really blessings in disguise, signs not to abandon your goals but to seek them in some different way? As I stumbled along my own road, I began to see the truth—stumbling blocks can be stepping-stones when they're viewed with the right frame of mind.

> *There are two ways to conquer adversity:*
> *We can change whatever is causing it, or*
> *we can change ourselves to move past it.*

Although there's no shortage of books that describe different ways to get healthy and fit, none has addressed, to a proper extent, the plight of the millions who've failed. This book is the first. It's unique in that while it challenges popular views about how to get fit, it guides you toward finding the "UFOs" (Unidentified Fitness Obstacles) that have kept you from reaching your goals.

This book is not for those who only have casual concerns for their health. It's for those who'd like to improve themselves and are making an honest effort but haven't progressed as much as they'd like and are stumped by their lack of success. It's for frustrated fitness enthusiasts whose workouts have failed to work out.

As opposed to providing one program that pretends to meet everyone's needs, this book helps you to expose fitness blocks that are *individually* based. Because it uncovers an obstacle's source instead of just dwelling on symptoms, it proposes the kind of strategic cures that can lead to *permanent* change. By learning how to identify your personal UFOs, you'll be able to find the missing links in your quest to be optimally fit.

At first, when I thought about writing this book, I felt a great deal of frustration. It disturbed me to see that so many people were finding it hard to get fit. Too often I saw them fall short of their goals without ever realizing why. Instead of addressing their failings, they were eager to find a quick fix. They wanted a magic formula that would "cure" them, once and for all.

It's time that we all face the truth. There is no *one* magic formula that will help us to get in shape. Because we all have different blocks, in addition to different goals, we can't use the same ingredients in our recipe for success. The "magic" lies in discovering what these ingredients actually are. The "formula" must be a personal one; there is truly no other way.

The process of getting ourselves in shape is much like solving a puzzle. Before we can hope to solve it, though, there are pieces that must be found. Consider your own fitness puzzle. In what ways is it unique? Are emotional conflicts keeping you from reaching your physical goals? Do you have any physical health concerns that you haven't exposed or addressed? Should you try a new way of training? Regardless of what your puzzle entails, it's one you'll be challenged to solve. The challenge, once you find the pieces, is to identify how they're all linked. It's because people rarely accept this and are impatient about their success, so that most, even as they strive to improve their health, keep shooting themselves in the foot. It's as if in their hurry to water their grass, they keep standing on top of the hose!

Part I of this book reveals what it means to get fit from the *inside out*. It gives you the basic framework for getting your body in sync with your mind. It shows you how to eliminate your old, self-defeating patterns, transcending your psychological blocks to realize your true potential. In addition, it serves as a guide to discovering new ways to lift your spirit, helping you find the insight you need to begin drawing strength from within. Last, it speaks to how UFOs can arise when we're too ego centered and how to avoid being influenced by deceptive, unhealthy ideals.

Part II gets more specific about what types of blocks are common and shows you how to address your personal mind/body UFOs. By completing simple checklists (to assess your UFO symptoms), you discover how mental and physical blocks can hinder your quest to get fit. Then, after looking at blocks that stem from emotional UFOs, you learn about common UFOs that have biochemical roots. In addition, you learn new ways to expose nutritional UFOs, in part by seeing how popular diet advice may be steering you wrong. Again, by completing self-tests to assess your specific symptoms, you're provided with tools that will help you make links to your own individual blocks.

Part III reveals the facts you should know about exercise UFOs. It begins by exposing obstacles that can result from misleading advice and challenges you to rethink your approach to becoming aerobically fit. It also discusses weight-training blocks that you may not know you have and offers unique new guidelines for reaching your muscular fitness potential. Last, you're given a simple plan to integrate what you learn. By identifying the UFOs that are personally most problematic, you learn, by hurdling *the right blocks first*, how to reach greater heights of success. As your profile unfolds, while objectively taking a look at what holds you back, you gain a whole new perspective both of yourself and about working out.

As you start to gain this perspective, you may have to confront certain fears. In the past, for example, I feared that my goals were impractical or far-fetched. So whenever I failed to reach them, I assumed I had proved myself right. Too often, though, the reason I failed was because I feared that I would. My fear was actually causing me to sabotage my success. In order to move beyond my fear, confronting it was the key. If I'd been unwilling to do so, I would never have reached my potential.

Our fears keep us from growing in ways that are critical to our success. The irony is that facing them is the only way they can be tamed. As long as we fail to do so, they'll continue to hold us back.

To illustrate, consider Jane's story. Jane was a client, thirty years old, who was struggling to stay in shape. At times she was very disciplined. She rarely missed a workout and appeared to be very fit. But other times she avoided the gym, gained weight, and became depressed.

When I asked Jane to explain this, she seemed to be at a loss. "It's when I start looking my best," Jane said, "that I always seem to derail. I don't know what it could possibly be that prevents me from staying on track. I'm sick of trying so hard all the time and having it be for naught. I'm tired of working so hard to lose weight and then always gaining it back."

As I listened to Jane talk more about her feelings regarding the process, it was clear she was being sabotaged by her unidentified fears. Whenever she looked and felt her best, she was praised for the way that she looked. She also received more attention, particularly from men. The result was that she felt vulnerable, or as she put it, "viewed as an object." In addition, she feared being envied, both by friends and by those at her gym. Though she wasn't entirely conscious of this, she responded by not working out. It was then that she started to overeat and subsequently, gained weight. Subconsciously, she held the belief that by looking less shapely and fit, she'd no longer have to be scrutinized, judged, or resented by envious peers.

This is just one example of how fear gets in the way. It's not always so complex. Sometimes we simply fear change. When this is true, we discount advice or refuse to try anything new. When the thought of a change makes us fear the worst, it can feel like too much of a risk. The fear of being criticized or of making a foolish choice can in and of itself become an obstacle to success. When this occurs, unknowingly, we keep setting ourselves up to fail. We may *think* that we're moving forward, and may trust that we're on the right track, but we don't often see as we step on the gas that we're also applying the brake!

The lesson here, and throughout this book, is one that gets right to the point: If you always do what you've always done, you'll get what you've always gotten. In other words, to be your best, be open to making a change. Open your eyes to see the things that are *really* in your way.

Open your mind to a new way to think, to challenge yourself in new ways. The success of your journey depends on it.

Whatever lies before me is not blocking my next step; it is my next step.

—MAUREEN BRADY

◆ **EXERCISE** ◆

Are Your Workouts Working Out?

Complete the following test. It will give you a sense of just how much you're affected by UFOs (Unidentified Fitness Obstacles). Put an **X** next to each statement that directly applies to you. The more that you find you relate to, the more you will gain from this book.

———— I do what I see lots of others do, but I don't get the same results.

———— I feel like I'm being limited by factors "beyond my control."

———— I rarely stick to a program for more than three or four weeks.

———— I'm enticed by every new gimmick or fad that I see advertised on TV (trendy exercise devices, "revolutionary" new diets, unorthodox approaches to exercise).

———— My efforts are too often manic: I frequently start a new program feeling hopeful and inspired, but often within a few days (or weeks) my interest tends to wane.

———— I'm obsessed with getting the inside track on the "best" kind of diet or workout, but I don't very often consider the ways that my mind is affecting my body.

———— I sense that there's something holding me back, but I'm not sure what it is.

———— It's hard for me to eat right and exercise at the same time: Usually if I succeed at one, it's at the expense of the other.

———— When something seems to be *working*, I'm compelled to do something new: I often feel tempted to stray from my path to look for a better course.

———— When something is clearly *not* working, I rarely consider a change: Even when I fall short of my goals, I refuse to try anything new.

—— Despite recurring injuries, I continue to train the same way: I keep doing things that are hurting me when it's obvious something is wrong.

—— My attitude toward working out is generally all or none: I must set and achieve the most challenging goals or I won't make an effort at all.

—— I believe that when the time is right, I'll be able to step up my efforts, that "one of these days" I'll finally be able to do what it takes to succeed.

—— My motivation to exercise *always* wanes in the winter (or fall).

—— My energy level varies in a fairly predictable pattern.

—— Only when I have specific goals do I train on a regular basis.

Scoring

1–2: *You're probably doing fairly well, except for a few common problems.* This book will still be of help to you, though, if these problems have not been resolved.

3–4: *Your progress is being impeded by some factors you need to address.* But you may not be far from achieving your goals—once you attend to your problem.

5–6: *Your results will be slight or impermanent if you stay on your current course.* Though you may see progress sporadically, it's likely to be short-lived.

7+: *You need more help than you realize.* There are clearly some things that you need to address that are very much in your way. Unless you learn how to identify and conquer your UFOs, you're likely to find that you always fail or struggle to reach your goals.

◆ ◆ ◆

PART I

Finding Inner Fitness

• • •

Laying the Foundation for a Body/Mind Connection

Mind-Sets

Connecting Your Mind to Your Body; Walking a Mindful Path

At every moment, our bodies are responding to messages from our minds. So what messages is your mind giving your body?

—Margo Adair

When I was twenty years old, I graduated from college. And not a moment too soon. After years of being preached to and told what I should do, I was tired of taking advice. I was finally ready to give it.

At the time, I could think of only one way to assume an advice-giving role: I'd use lots of jargon, big fancy words, and intricate, technical terms. That way, people would be impressed and more apt to follow my lead. I was eager to make a name for myself, to become well known in my field, to be worshiped and praised by a legion of fans sporting frocks that said, "Body by Mike." "Now that I have a degree," I thought, "my knowledge will be respected. People will value my wisdom. They'll believe everything that I say."

I couldn't have been more naive. I soon found out that some people knew (or thought they knew) more than me. To my dismay, there were few who had much faith in my advice.

"I bet they'll respect me more," I thought, "if I speak with more conviction." So I did. "Brothers and sisters!" I shouted, "I've come to save your souls! Bring me your love handles, saddlebags, and unsightly, dimple-plagued thighs! Come, atone for your evil sins and your idle, sluggardly ways! Surrender your flab-laden figures. *It's never too late to be saved!*

Strangely, my sermon, glib as it was, primarily fell on deaf ears. But I didn't let it upset me. "It's only a matter of time," I thought, "before they accept my advice. Then, as soon as they follow it, they'll see that it really works!"

What happened made my prediction look like it couldn't have been more wrong. People did follow my guidance, but something still wasn't quite right. For some inexplicable reason, they were still falling short of their goals.

At the time, I was blind to the fact that what I was witnessing happens a lot. Most people who try to exercise fail to attain their goals or maintain them. Why is this so often true? Because physical fitness is seldom achieved by focusing just on the body. In order to reach our fitness goals, and maintain them for the long term, we must overcome the *emotional* blocks that consistently get in our way. We must be concerned with the state of our mind, not just the state of our body.

This is a notion we tend to dismiss when we think about getting more fit. We've been led to believe that getting in shape is strictly a physical process. We've been told that diet and exercise are the only true paths to success. But the link between our body and mind is stronger than we can imagine. In fact, it's seeing (and making) this link that frees us to be fully fit. It's by doing so that we'll more clearly see, and avoid, what is holding us back.

This chapter reveals how your thoughts and beliefs can affect what goes on in your body. It helps you discover new ways to eliminate old, self-defeating patterns, by giving you simple, straightforward techniques for becoming more self-aware. By learning how "thought-field therapy" helps to reprogram old patterns of thought, you'll see how this leading-edge tool can be used to eliminate common blocks. You'll learn how to break through the energy blocks that keep you from finding success.

Self-Sabotage

When we fail to achieve our fitness goals, we're often full of excuses: a busy schedule, obligations, factors beyond our control. No matter what the reason is we usually find something to blame. The truth, though, is that when we fail, we tend to blame the wrong things. More often than not, our tendency is to sabotage ourselves.

Why is this so often true? Perhaps it's because in reality, a lot of us question our mettle. We doubt that we really have what it takes to stay on the path to success. Too often, this negative mind-set becomes a self-fulfilling prophesy. It's why we can't help but falter and why we so often give up.

Consider Michelle's story. Although she had often tried to lose weight, she experienced little success. She was afraid that if she tried again, the result would be much the same. She was also afraid she'd be criticized, much like she'd been in the past.

"It's no use," said Michelle. "I'll never be in good shape. My friends all think that I'm hopeless; in fact, they tell me I'll never lose weight. They say that when hell freezes over, if I'm lucky, I'll drop a few pounds.

"I wish I could diet," she went on to say, "but for some reason, I just can't. It seems like whenever I try, I always end up losing control. That's when my boyfriend usually starts making comments about how I look. The worst part is that the more he does, the more I want to eat. He says he's trying to motivate me, but it doesn't help at all."

Michelle had problems besides the abuse that she took from her boyfriend and friends. Her use of over-the-counter drugs had been getting out of control. "I tried using laxatives," she said, "but they just made me sick. Now I'm taking diet pills. All I know is I won't work out until I lose some weight. There's no way that I can go to a gym, not while I look like this!"

By projecting her fear of criticism on her boyfriend and her friends, Michelle, without even realizing it, was inviting their hurtful replies. To cope with the way that they made her feel, she usually overate. Consequently, she gained more weight and began to use more drugs. In effect, her coping responses were actually serving to fuel her fear.

Michelle's conditioned reflex was to sabotage herself. She was repeating familiar patterns, not because they made sense, but because they were what she was comfortable with and all she had ever known. To understand why this happened, she needed to be more conscious. She had to expose the emotional blocks that were dictating how she behaved. Only then could she conquer her fears and begin to achieve her goals.

In various ways, we all do things to sabotage our success. As you recall, Jane became anxious when people *admired* how she looked. When she finally began to acknowledge her fear, she was able to see the truth. Although on a conscious level she was starved for attention and praise, down deep, on a subconscious level, she had a much stronger need to feel safe. For Jane, being safe meant not being ogled or envied by critical peers. Once she perceived how her fears played out and affected the way she behaved, she was finally able to stop doing things that prevented her long-term success.

As you look at many people's lives, you see that their suffering is in a way gratifying, for they are comfortable in it. They make their lives a living hell, but a familiar one.

—RAM DASS

Emotional Conflicts: Barriers to Achieving Physical Fitness?

Why is getting in shape so often such an elusive goal? What is the root, or most common cause, of recurrent fitness failure? As psychologists delve even deeper into the link between body and mind, what they are finding, time and again, essentially comes down to this: Physical blocks result from conflicts rooted in our emotions.

According to William Whisenant, Ph.D., in his book *Psychological Kinesiology*, "There is an intimate interaction between emotional and physical functioning." It's emotional conflicts, he says, that portend our destructive reflexes. They're a trigger for the behaviors that repeatedly cause us to fail.

Some of us think that by getting in shape, these conflicts will disappear. For example, we think that losing weight will bolster our self-esteem. But often we feel even less secure the more we invest in the process. Deep-seated conflicts come to the fore that keep us from reaching our goals. Examples are unresolved childhood wounds or questions about our self-worth. These conflicts are much like banana peels that keep showing up in our path. Unless we start finally picking them up, they're apt to keep making us slip.

Often, resolving these conflicts is simply a matter of making them known. But it's not always quite so simple. At times, it isn't enough that we reveal the root of our struggle. In fact, when we do and we *still* feel stuck, we may have to delve even deeper. To find out exactly what stands in our way, we may need to be more open-minded.

The first time I opened my own mind, what I found took me quite by surprise. Although I had heard about energy fields and how they relate to our body, the notion that they were in fact very real was one I found hard to accept. But once I observed the response people had to a new kind of energy therapy, I started to wonder if, possibly, there was more to all this than I thought. Suddenly, I was intrigued enough to take a more in-depth look.

We are what we think. All that we are arises with our thoughts. With our thoughts, we make our world.

—BUDDHA

Thought-Field Therapy

Clinical psychologist Roger Callahan, Ph.D., is the creator of thought-field therapy (TFT), a means to correct imbalances involving the body's "energy systems." These systems consist of specific, tangible pathways (or channels) of energy that, like electronic circuitry, run in patterns all over our body. It's the data we store in our "thought-field," Dr. Callahan dares to suggest, that open (or close) these channels, or in a sense, are what "program" these circuits. The thought-field, he says, is the place where we hold our innate and conditioned beliefs. It's the place where we form the patterns that shape and control how we feel and behave.

For some of you this concept may be difficult to conceive. You might even question its emphasis in a book about fitness and health. But if as you start to read about this you're able to keep your mind open, its significance should become clear to you with regard to becoming more fit. You'll begin to see how energy blocks can be exercise blocks as well.

Callahan claims that when our thoughts are negative or disturbing, it blocks or disrupts our circuitry, causing an energy imbalance. This negative information is called a *perturbation*. Perturbations are the catalysts for our self-defeating behaviors. They trigger the mind and body events that keep us from reaching our goals.

To put this idea in a simpler way, consider this example: If you believe you cannot lose weight, you may have a perturbation. When a thought-field is disrupted by (or is "holding") a perturbation, the energy paths in your body will either be blocked or in disarray. Callahan calls this phenomenon *psychological reversal*. It's when we're reversed, he claims, that we do things that are in contrast to our conscious desires and goals. An example of this is a person who says he wants to improve his health but continues to eat unhealthy foods, or continues to overeat.

When you're struggling (or failing) to get in shape, a reversal is often the cause. Reversals affect your mind in ways that have much to do with your body. What does this really mean? It means that your body's resistance to change may be caused by a state of reversal. It means that a state of reversal can also be physiologic.

People who are reversed are prone to focusing on what's wrong. Instead of noting successes, they obsess about how they've failed. They tend to dwell on what *hasn't* occurred as opposed to on what has. For example, "I *only* lost ten pounds," instead of, "I lost five pounds!" If you think this sounds a lot like you, you'll want to consider what follows.

Testing for Psychological Reversal

If as you strive to get in shape, you consistently find it a struggle, it's likely that part of the problem is that you're psychologically reversed. But if you require some proof of this, this simple test should help.

1. Hold one arm out straight to the side, parallel to the floor.
2. Have someone place his or her hand on your lower arm or around you wrist.

3. Imagine yourself feeling anxious about an issue of great concern. Close your eyes and imagine you're having a weight-loss-related problem (for example, food cravings or bingeing or whatever comes promptly to mind). Focus *intently* on negative thoughts and feelings around this subject.

4. Now by lifting your straight arm up against your partner's hand, apply as much force as you can while saying (out loud) "I want to lose weight" (or whatever you'd like to accomplish). Your partner should note how much force you apply while resisting your maximum effort.

5. Relax your arm for at least ten seconds.

6. Now repeat this procedure (with the same arm, in the same way), but this time while making a statement like "I'm happy the way I am." If your partner notes that you use more force while making the latter statement, then with regard to losing weight, you are in fact reversed.

The results of this test are quite telling in the majority of cases. But for clearer or more objective results, you can use a dynamometer (a tool for measuring strength). When you squeeze it, it measures the gripping force that you can apply with your hand. A chiropractor may have this device or others that work the same way.

It's often been my experience that people don't know they're reversed. I've also found that reversals can be at the root of a whole host of problems. Some examples include athletes who are in slumps or whose play is subpar, or chronic yo-yo dieters who keep losing and gaining back weight. I'm convinced that it's when we're in this state that we tend to experience setbacks. I believe it explains, in large part, why our efforts are often in vain.

Learning to Break Through Energy Blocks: Correcting a State of Reversal

While TFT is the best way I know to treat and correct a reversal, it's also a very effective means to address more specific problems. It largely involves using energy points, eye movements, and affirmations in problem-specific patterns tailored to overcome personal blocks. Callahan calls these patterns, or treatment sequences, *algorithms*. Callahan's work with these treatments has produced astounding results. He's found that by "tapping" strategically located energy points on the body, meridians (channels of energy) that have been blocked can be rapidly cleared. When using the right eye movements, sequence of tapping, and affirmations, a powerful energy shift can occur that corrects a state of imbalance. The tapping works in a way that's akin to tripping a circuit breaker. In a sense, when you activate relevant points to rectify an imbalance, it's like you are reconnecting a broken electrical circuit. By repeating the affirmations, you reinforce the connection.

Depending on what the block is, a treatment approach can vary, and an energy treatment sequence can involve quite a few different points. I'm amazed by how well and how often thought-field therapy tends to work, even for those who are skeptics or who have very stubborn blocks. I've never encountered a faster means to eliminate fitness constraints.

I was once approached by a middle-aged man who told me he lacked motivation. He said that he wanted to get in shape but could not seem to stay on track. "I don't know why it is," Bob said, "but I'm rarely inspired to work out. It seems like the more that I need to, the less I usually want to. I also have very strong cravings for unhealthy, fat-laden foods. When I do, it's usually hard for me to resist the temptation to binge. I can't ever seem to help myself. Why does this always happen?"

My instincts told me to test Bob to see if he was reversed. First I asked him to lift his arm up hard against my hand. While he did this, I asked him to say out loud, "I want to continue to train." Then he applied force again while saying, "I want to control how I eat."

It was at this point that I asked Bob to say, "I want to stay like I am." It was then that, much to *his* surprise but not so much to mine, he was actually able to raise his arm with a greater amount of force. While his conscious mind was telling him "you should eat less and exercise more," his subconscious was telling him not to, that his efforts were destined to fail.

Once Bob's reversal was treated, he could hardly believe the change. His anxiety level rapidly dropped and his energy level increased. From then on, when he felt lazy or inclined to overeat, he was actually able to shift his thoughts by repeating his treatment sequence. The result? He rarely missed a workout, lost more than thirty pounds, and was able to get into better shape than he ever imagined he could.

Unlike energy treatments that either work slowly or don't work at all, thought-field therapy tends to work fast and accomplishes lasting results. In addition, results can be measured; it works in tangible ways. With a rate of success that studies reveal exceeds 95 percent, TFT is a treatment approach that truly lives up to its promise. Even if you remain skeptical, I suggest that you give it a try. You've got nothing to lose by doing so, and you're apt to be glad that you did.

Because I didn't invent TFT, I can't tell you more than I have. By contacting Dr. Callahan, though, you can access the info you need. In addition, finding a therapist should not be a difficult task. Thought-field therapists often are found through alternative health publications. (To locate appropriate resources, refer to the Appendix.)

Every thought you think, every belief you hold becomes a bio-chemical reality in your body. Any persistent symptom is your inner wisdom trying to bring your attention to an area that needs compassion.

—CHRISTIANE NORTHRUP, M.D.

The Role of Psychotherapy in Caring for the Body

Although I often propose the idea of therapy to my clients, I don't very often get a response that isn't in some way defensive. Mainly it's something like, "What do you mean? Do you really think I'm *that* bad?" Some say it's only for "troubled souls" or "mostly a waste of time." I've also been told that therapists are only "expensive friends," or that people need counseling only if they're "desperate, ill, or weak."

As I see it, this way of thinking couldn't be any more off the mark. In no way should those who seek counseling be thought of as desperate, ill, or weak. On the contrary, asking for help requires a tremendous amount of courage. This courage comes from a place of strength, *not* from a place of weakness.

Perhaps you, too, would benefit from reframing your point of view.

How about thinking of therapy as an adjunct to getting in shape? You could even think of a therapist as a "personal coach for your mind." Therapy isn't only for those who feel that they've hit rock bottom. Conversely, it's a proactive means of uncovering unconscious blocks. It's an investment in oneself. The right type of psychotherapy can provide you with insight you lack. It can reveal how emotional obstacles may be keeping you from getting fit.

Counseling can help you physically as much as it can emotionally. It can help you find out what the "real" reasons are that you're struggling to get in good shape. They may actually be quite different from what you've been led to believe. You may find, for example, that your primary goal is *not* to improve your health. It may be, instead, to impress someone or perhaps to impress yourself. You may also find that by trying so hard to create an attractive facade, you're masking a problem with low self-esteem or a low-grade state of depression. If this is the case, working out won't work, at least not well, for long. If you think that this doesn't apply to you, you may need to face the truth. If you've failed to achieve your fitness goals, a new workout may not be the answer. And if you've been finding it hard to lose weight, the problem may not be your diet. Instead, you may need to consider the ways that your mind is affecting your body.

Over time, as I learned even more about ways that the body and mind are connected, I realized that it would benefit me to expand my professional training. At first, when I thought about different ways to further my education, my plan was simply to work toward another fitness-related degree. But I came to see that this wasn't the most beneficial route I could take. When forced to concede that my fitness advice was limited in its scope, I decided to seek a graduate degree in the field of mental health. It was then that I stopped seeing working out as purely a physical process. I realized that most fitness obstacles must be addressed from the *inside out*. When this becomes more apparent to *you*, you may see your priorities change. You may, for example, decide that you want to set more forgiving goals. When you do, you may find that the negative thoughts that have hindered your efforts will ebb, helping you move past stubborn blocks that have kept you from getting more fit. I refer to these blocks as UFOs, or Unidentified Fitness Obstacles. UFOs are the missing links in your quest for a better body. They're the things that nobody talks about, the things that are most in your way.

They're the spiritual, mental, and physical blocks that keep you from staying on track—for example, a low-grade depression, problems with sleep, or SAD, or even a common food allergy, hormone imbalance, or low self-esteem. These are just some of the obvious blocks that are rarely, if ever, suspected. They're the things, as this book will help you to see, that are most apt to thwart your success.

> *I see a therapist every other hour. Some people say, "That's too much therapy." And I say, "You go to hell." Because I've got a lot of anger.*
>
> —CONAN O'BRIEN

The Mood Journal

Therapy isn't the only means to connect with your subconscious mind. Using a private "mood journal" also can be of tremendous help. Keeping a written record of your thoughts and the ways you feel can help to reveal old patterns that have kept you from reaching your goals.

A journal can help you to process your fitness-related feelings. Whether they are about dieting or about problems involving your health, these feelings must be expressed and released in an ongoing, tangible way. As your story unfolds, and your journal becomes a new way to vent how you feel, you may find that a certain issue has repeatedly been of concern. This sudden glimpse of reality may help you to see things in a much different way. It may give you a clearer view of how you can conquer your UFOs.

Writing down thoughts and feelings is beneficial to our health, says James Pennebaker, a professor of psychology at the University of Texas. Over a period of several months (while at Southern Methodist University), Pennebaker asked his students to write in detail about college life. As his students expressed on paper their fears and concerns about daily life, he found that in most of their cases, they became more resistant to stress. Surprisingly, he observed evidence that their immune function had improved.

The results of this study are clear: Writing about thoughts and feelings can produce physiological change. If you're struggling to reach your fitness goals, it's important to keep this in mind.

Finding Your Best "Workout Zone": Attaining a Focused, Centered State of Spirit, Mind, and Body

Exercise. Some folks contend that if it's not fun, it's not something we're going to do. I'm not sure this is true. I don't agree that exercise must necessarily be fun. A better word is "rewarding." While exercise certainly *can* be fun, it can be many other things too. In fact, it can help to enhance your mood or help to alleviate stress. There are many ways besides having fun to benefit from working out.

For most of us, though, there are too many times when we're not benefiting at all; when we basically go through the motions and feel as if training is simply a chore. If instead of working out mindlessly we could learn to connect with our body, we'd find ourselves feeling more energized and inspired about what we do. We'd look forward to feeling the "high" that results when we train in a mindful manner.

To channel our energy properly, our mind must be tuned to our body. This means that we must pay attention to how an exercise *feels*. People who know how to focus can appreciate how this works. In fact, they often develop a sort of physical ESP (*ESP*, in this case, meaning *exercise*-sensory perception). They know that to do an exercise well, they must resonate with each movement, as if they're striking a chord that says, "This is the right thing to do." As a result, they always ensure that their movements are smooth and precise. They always attend to the details regarding position and proper technique. They respect their limitations—they're attuned to what serves them best.

By focusing on the proper form and rhythm of a movement, you'll achieve a state, a "zone" if you will, in which your efforts will thrive. As a result, you'll have greater strength as well as much better endurance. Instead of fighting your body, you'll be giving it what it needs. You'll understand the importance of having your body in sync with your mind.

When we perform our workouts mindfully (meaning focused, and in our zone), I believe we draw strength from our *spirit* as much as we do from our pecs or our quads. In fact, to this day, whenever I train, I attempt to tap into this spirit. I think of this spirit as energy that is centered or stored deep within. The way I try to access it is by picturing it in my mind. As I start to contract my muscles, I imagine this energy spreading, feeding my muscles with "high-octane fuel" that will boost my endurance and strength. The results of this are profound. I feel like I'm being energized by a powerful inner force. Because of this, I can perform in a way that before doing this I could not.

Some people claim that to visualize actually helps to reprogram our thoughts. Positive visual images, they say, create physiologic changes, including more strength, more energy, and an improved blood flow to our muscles. If you decide to try this, and you find that it serves you well, you may want to use visualization as an adjunct to your routine, whether it's while you're training or as a warm-up before you work out.

> *The difficulty is to learn to perceive with your whole body, not just with your eyes and reason. You must train your body to make it a good receptor. The body is an awareness; and it must be treated impeccably.*
>
> —CARLOS CASTANEDA

Using Self-Hypnosis for a Healthy "Physical" Mind-Set

There is no special secret to performing self-hypnosis. It doesn't require any complex skill, and it's not a mysterious trick. It's really very simple. Essentially, self-hypnosis is focused relaxation. It's a way to condition your body to respond to the state of your mind.

There are many techniques that you can use to relax your body and mind. One that works especially well is progressive relaxation. You start by imagining part of your body becoming increasingly heavy, so heavy that it cannot be moved, no matter how hard you try. It's usually best to begin at your feet and to slowly work your way up. For example, you might imagine at first that your feet feel like big blocks of lead. By imagining them feeling heavier (as they "sink" slowly into the floor), the tension will drain from your muscles and joints, and your feet will begin to relax. As you move on to other body parts (for example, your legs and your arms), try to imagine each part of your body becoming increasingly heavy (and getting progressively heavier as you become more and more relaxed). When your entire body is fully relaxed, you can start making affirmations.

You may also choose to tense and relax your muscles, one at a time, or to relax your body by practicing deep, steady, focused breaths. It doesn't matter so much what you do, nor does it matter much how, as long as whatever you do consistently works and is not too involved. When your body and mind are quiet, you've succeeded in setting the stage; you've created an optimum climate for envisioning your success.

Healthy Affirmations for Optimum Physical Fitness

As we strive to improve our body, some resistance is bound to arise. We may find, in fact, that our own inner judge has a big, blunt, and very loud mouth. Too often, it gives us the message that "We can't, we won't, and we aren't." That's why affirmations can often be such a valuable tool. They're especially good for drowning out our critical inner voice. When affirmations are properly used, consistently, over time, our old, self-defeating reflexes can be reprogrammed and even dispelled.

When you combine affirmation with imagery, it's especially effective. If, for example, you want to lose weight, you imagine yourself both looking and feeling exactly the way you desire. You would then repeat (as often as needed) the appropriate affirmations. Examples of affirmations are "I'm losing weight," "My body responds well to exercise," and "I'm developing a lean, healthy body." Although you can try to memorize them, you might want to put them on tape. Then you can play them back to yourself at the time and place that is best. By listening to a tape of the affirmations you prefer, you won't be concerned about missing words, or recalling them in the wrong way. In addition, a background of soft, peaceful music can help you relax with more ease.

It's best if you try not to focus too hard or be too concerned with the process. Imagine that you already are whatever you most want to be. Make sure, though, that your affirmations are always very specific. They should be about what you *are* doing as opposed to what you aren't, for example, "I *am* losing weight" as opposed to "I won't fail to lose weight."

When making affirmations, your choice of words is key. Be sure to keep them positive and to use the present tense, for example, "I *am* succeeding" instead of "I hope to achieve my goals." Flood your mind with self-talk that is positive and inspiring. Make that inner critic an advocate for your success.

Health/Fitness Affirmations

I deserve success.

I accept myself exactly the way I am.

I am (focused, disciplined, motivated).

I am committed to my success.

I am patient with myself as I (get in shape, lose weight).

I am (losing weight, gaining strength, improving my body, etc.).

My body responds well to exercise.

I feel (strong, empowered, energized) when I exercise.

I am persevering.

I am developing a (lean, healthy, defined, shapely, well-proportioned, muscular) body.

I respect myself and my body.

I understand and accept that (getting in shape, losing weight) is a process.

I (enjoy, appreciate, respect) the process.

My goal *is* the process.

The Goal Should Be the Process

Whenever people tell me that they *need* to get in shape, it's hard for me to be confident that they actually ever will. I'm convinced that this type of statement only sets them up to fail. I hear it most often when they're feeling desperate or pressured to make a big change. The inference is that they *must* get in shape, lest something bad occur. Rarely does this way of thinking help to create an inspired frame of mind.

Rather than think that we *should* or that we *need* to get in shape, we should try to adopt a mind-set that comes more from a place of strength. Instead, it's best to think more in terms of *wanting* to get in shape. It's when we attach the word "need" to things that we get hung up on results. The need to accomplish results or goals can actually become an obsession. And it's when we obsess about setting goals that we find them most hard to achieve.

To put this in perspective, imagine you're learning to skate. At first, while you're still learning, occasionally you may fall. If you're too hung up on the goal, for example, being a "perfect" skater, falling might upset your confidence to a greater extent than it should. Instead of viewing it simply as a normal part of the process, you may assume that you don't have the knack or won't ever be able to learn. Hence, you may become hard on yourself and be critical of your attempts. You may even abandon your efforts before you achieve success.

If you choose to quit after only one or even a number of falls, you rob yourself of a perfect chance to learn from your mistakes. The truth is that when learning to skate, falling is part of the process. And when your goal is to get in shape, so is missing a workout.

I once heard some politician say that "a goal is a dream with a deadline." It's my view, though, that for most fitness goals, deadlines are counterproductive. Although they can help in the short term, in the long run they can be harmful. Oftentimes, when we pressure ourselves to accomplish a time-constrained goal, we feel compelled to do ill-advised things that turn out to be very costly. Starving ourselves or relying on drugs are examples of what I mean.

With a sound and forgiving mind-set, goal setting serves us well. But when achieving goals is our focus, we can set ourselves up to fail. Why? Because if we obsess about reaching goals, we're apt to view slips as *slides*. If we ever hope to attain success, we must change our point of view. If instead we start to view getting in shape as an ongoing, personal *process*, we'll no longer feel compelled to pursue superficial, short-term goals. We'll be less concerned with *what* we achieve and more concerned with *how*. We'll refuse to see slipping as sliding. We see it as par for the course.

> *It is good to have an end to journey toward, but it is the journey that matters in the end.*
>
> —URSULA LEGUIN

Lifting Your Spirit

Putting Your Heart into Working Out; Making a Spiritual Connection

Each soul is a different shape. No one sees or feels your life the same way that you do. The secret to all tranquillity exists within your heart.

—John O'Donahue

The road to good health can be venturesome. It can lead us down many paths. Sadly, though, very few of them ever lead where we expect. How, then, can we be certain that we're traveling down the right path? How can we know, for sure, that we've selected the straightest course?

In my quest to improve my own health, I've come to acknowledge this: The paths that are truly best for me are invariably those with a *heart*. They're always paths that inspire me, paths in which I have faith. And as I look back, I can also see that they're always found within.

How can a path be found within? And what's the connection to getting in shape? To me, it's about tuning into the "voice" or the instinct that comes from our body. It's about trusting our intuition and accessing our inner guide, that part of us that knows what's best for our body as well as our mind. When we do, we see beyond our fears to a place where our course is clear. It's *there* that we find our pathway to optimum physical health.

This chapter offers the guidance you need to begin drawing strength from within. By learning simple, practical ways to discover your inner voice, you learn how to gain a palpable sense of your "spiritual fitness" needs. Also in this chapter, the following questions are posed: Can strengthening your spirit help you to accept and respect your body? Can you increase your physical strength by borrowing strength from within? Why is it such a struggle for you to get yourself into shape? Why are you so resistant to doing whatever it takes to succeed?

The answers to all of these questions can be found by trusting your heart, by putting some stock in your instinct for what will encourage and *fuel* you the most. Once you start trusting your instincts and tuning into the way that you feel, the way you'll begin to approach getting fit will in many ways change for the best. Instead of pursuing shallow goals, you'll start setting goals that make sense. You'll accept yourself more, judge yourself less, and compare yourself less to others. You might even give up your ego and, as a result, become more self-assured. In fact, you may find as you do so, and in time, gain a different perspective, that your ego is what has been keeping you from pursuing a mindful path.

It's when we are ego driven that we fail to honor the process. It's our ego that often compels us to make irresponsible choices. It invites compulsive behavior and the pursuit of impractical goals. It also narrows our focus. We forget about how we're affected on a mental and spiritual level. We become so focused on how we look that we forget how we feel. And so we repeatedly falter, oblivious to this void, looking outside of ourselves for something to kindle our dwindling fire. The truth, though, is that this fire *won't last* unless it is stoked from within. It must be ignited and fed in a way that's attuned to the path of your heart. But first you must learn to connect with it, and then to interpret its "language."

Tapping Your Physical Instincts

What is the language of your heart? Is it one you can understand? How does it speak to you, here and now, about everything that you've just read? Does it tell you it might be important? Or does it tell you it's not? You should seek and follow your own truth, as opposed to anything else. This doesn't mean that you have to ignore everything that you read or hear. It means that you should trust the part of yourself that knows what's best for *you*. It means that, ultimately, you are your own best guide.

To further decode this language, it will help to consider this: Whatever it is that excites you most, and connects you most with your soul, is not just the language you understand best but also the one you best hear. Think about it. What kinds of things have you done in your life that inspired you most of all, that have made you feel, in that moment, that nothing could ever be better? These are the things you must focus on, to connect with what calls you to action. When you learn how to *feel* this energy, and to understand how it is tapped, you're likely to find that it's just what you need to stay focused on challenging tasks. Like working out. Or eating well. Or achieving your physical goals. By finding that *passion* you'll lift your spirit to reach your fitness potential.

Consider Shirley's story. Shirley was a heavyset, middle-aged woman who'd been overweight most of her life. She'd been working out hard for several years but experienced little success. Regardless, she kept on trying. She believed she had no choice. She was told that being overweight was a serious risk to her health.

Shirley didn't mince words when it came to her feelings about working out. "My heart just isn't in it," she said. "It's boring and it hurts! I'm not inspired like others are. To me, it's nothing but work!"

Although it was clear how Shirley felt, I proceeded to question her further. "What is it," I asked, "that excites you most, that always brings you joy? What makes you feel like you could do whatever you set your mind to? Is there one thing you can think of that always lifts your spirits?"

"I really love gospel music," she said. "It seems to awaken my soul! I feel like a spirit moves me, like I'm being divinely inspired! Whenever I hear that music, I suddenly feel more alive!"

"How would it be," I replied, "if you were able to bottle that feeling? What if you could capture it and take it to the gym? What would it take to focus it and to use it when working out?"

Shirley then had a brainstorm. "If I went to the gym with my Walkman," she said, "I could exercise listening to gospel! I'm not sure if it'll help me, but it's certainly worth a try!"

Shirley's plan proved to be perfect. The music was just what she needed. It changed her entire attitude and approach toward working out. No longer did Shirley feel listless when it was time to go to the gym. From this point on, to her surprise, she *looked forward* to working out.

◆ EXERCISE ◆

Tools You Can Use to Enhance the Way You Experience Working Out

Choose three "tools" from the following list and add two more of your own. List them in order of preference and then expand them to be more specific (for example, next to your favorite music, list the specific artists, songs, and music styles that you prefer). Now examine your personal list of workout-enhancing tools. Can you see how you might use them to breathe new life into your routine?

—— Walkman

—— Your favorite music

—— Television

—— Inspirational videos (sporting events, exercise tapes, action films)

—— A tape of inspiring musical selections

—— Workout attire that is fun to wear and flattering to your shape (in a comfortable style, a perfect fit, soft fabric, or favorite color)

—— State-of-the-art exercise equipment

—— Comfortable, lightweight footwear

_____

_____

◆ ◆ ◆

Oftentimes, when I exercise, I listen to sound tracks from Rocky. *If I'm ever feeling too tired to train, or I'm not really in the mood, playing those tapes is just what I need to get in the right frame of mind. They never fail to pick me up—I always find them inspiring.*

—RON

What do you think is the key, then, to enhancing the way *you* work out? Regardless of whether it's finding your best way to train or getting inspired, the key is connecting your heart to your mind as well as your mind to your body. One man I knew bought a big-screen TV and set it up in his home gym. In front of it, he placed a rowing machine, a treadmill, and a bike. He loved to follow professional sports, football in particular. So whenever a game was scheduled, he gathered a few of his friends not only to watch the football game but also so they could work out. They looked forward to getting together like this and sharing their passion for sports. And while they worked out, that passion was what would enhance and inspire their efforts.

In order to be inspired, you don't always have to go anywhere or rely on any one thing. You simply need to find a way for your passions to spring to life. Think back to a memorable incident or to a once-in-a-lifetime event. Remember a time you felt energized and like things could never be better! By recalling these types of feelings, right before you begin to work out, you'll be primed to approach whatever you do in a much more spirited way. By doing this, you'll warm up your heart *before* warming up your body.

> *Before I begin to exercise, I like to prepare my mind. So while I'm on the mat stretching, or warming up on the bike, I'll close my eyes and remember a time when something I did brought me joy. Sometimes, I think about sporting events that for me were a special thrill. Other times, I'll try to recall how I felt on a special occasion. It's memories like these that connect me with feelings I almost forgot that I had. Feeling these feelings inspires me and gets me excited about working out.*
>
> —NORMAN

Learning to Trust Your Heart

Maybe this notion of trusting your heart is hard for you to accept. Perhaps to you it seems whimsical or even a bit far-fetched. You may even doubt that you have a heart, at least in the spiritual sense. But if you have ever been moved or inspired by a feeling you couldn't explain, you probably wouldn't argue if someone inferred that it came from your heart. To follow your heart, essentially, means tuning into the way you feel. Your heart is the place where you'll find your best motivation to work out.

If you're still not convinced that you'll gain anything by making a mind-heart connection, here is a point to consider that may sell you on the idea: The more that you're able to do so, the more you'll accept your body. You'll see that the way you *look* depends in large part on how you *feel*. By being *less* body focused, you'll actually have *more* success.

Granted, some people who are body focused *do* achieve some success. Their success, though, tends to be fleeting and rarely lives up to its promise. The results they achieve aren't likely to last and can cost them their long-term health. Consider your own experience. If you train too often, diet too strictly, or use drugs to perfect your physique, all that you're going to experience is a rise prior to your fall. This is like planting a bomb on yourself and hoping it never explodes! The only way to defuse it is by being true to yourself—rejecting the myth of perfection and letting go of your need to conform. But in order for you to do this, you must build your spiritual strength.

It's important to have a strong spirit in order to thrive in a self-conscious world. It gives us permission to be okay with simply being ourselves. Without any urge to compare or compete, we can follow our own best course. By accepting our faults and shortcomings, we can let go of our expectations. Then when we stop *expecting* some kind of perfect result, we begin to let go of the hang-ups that are limiting our success.

> *The curious paradox is, that when we accept ourselves exactly the way we are, only then can we change.*
>
> —CARL ROGERS

When we fail to respond to our efforts, it's a cry from our inner voice. It's urging us to respect ourselves and then to rethink our goals. One such goal that many of us have is to be what we're told is "ideal." We may tell ourselves that "ideal isn't real," but for some reason we don't listen. We disregard our inner voice and ignore our inner wisdom.

How can we make sure we hear it? By creating the time and space for ourselves to gain distance from daily distractions. Whether it's singing, dancing, painting, reading, writing, or just plain playing, we need to make time for our passions as well as our simplest pleasures. When we do, we'll see that the road to good health is found when we're living our truth. It's when we begin to recognize this that we'll stop falling short of our goals. Instead of being so hard on ourselves and feeling so out of control, we'll learn to be more self-accepting *and* more able to go with the flow.

> *Spontaneity is the heart of all spirituality. Anything that is deliberate or forced damages the spiritual sense. The soul is shy and oblique; it has its own natural rhythm. When we manage to let go of our programs and their forced intensities, we come into an ease with ourselves. The soul delights when we allow ourselves to connect with our deeper nature.*
>
> —JOHN O'DONAHUE

◆ EXERCISE ◆

Fitness-Related Activities That Favor a Heart, Mind, and Body Connection

Put a check next to the things on this list that you think you'd enjoy the most. Then add three of your own to the list and arrange them in order of preference. Now expand the list to include some specifics about each choice (for example, volleyball at the YMCA, blading with friends in the park). Can you think of any additional ways to expand on some of your options?

—— Dancing

—— Competitive team sports (e.g., basketball, soccer, hockey)

—— Individual sports (cycling, running, rowing)

—— Swimming

—— Skiing

—— Volleyball

—— Power walking

—— Boxing (aerobic, speed, or heavy bag)

—— Tai chi

—— Yoga

—— Aerobics (dance, box, jazz, funk)

—— Water/aqua aerobics

—— Ice-skating

—— Roller-skating

—— In-line skating

—— Hiking/backpacking

—— Training for competition (sports, road races, bodybuilding, powerlifting, triathlons, biathlons, swim meets)

—— Cross-country skiing

_____

_____

_____

◆ ◆ ◆

◆ EXERCISE ◆

Inspiring Exercise Environments

From the following list, put a check next to five of the places you enjoy most. Then add two of your own to the list and arrange them in order of preference. Be as specific as possible about locations and events (for example, riding your bike on a trail that passes through mountains or woods). In what ways might you fit these things into your daily routine?

—— Beach

—— Mountain trails

—— Woods

—— Country roads

—— Parks

—— National forests

—— Wildlife reserves

—— Ponds, lakes, or rivers

—— A bare-bones, no-frills, hard-core gym

—— An upscale, modern, fully equipped fitness center

—— A small, intimate, hometown health club

—— A private home gym

—— In front of a window or on a deck overlooking the ocean, mountains, etc.

—— Your old high school or college athletic fields

—— High school or college weight room

—— Basketball court

—— Hockey rink

—— Roller rink

—— A memorable/nostalgic location or route

—— Your old neighborhood or "stomping grounds"

—— A location/setting like one in a favorite/inspirational movie (*Rocky*/Philadelphia, *Pumping Iron*/Gold's Gym)

—— A health/fitness vacation (fitness cruise, spa, ranch)

_____

_____

◆ ◆ ◆

"Exorcising" Your Ego

Breaking Through Ego Barriers

It's better to look good, than to feel good.

—Billy Crystal

As Wilma gets in the checkout line at the Bedrock Stop & Shop, her eyes are instantly drawn to the rack of popular magazines. "Hey Betty," she whispers softly, doing her best to avoid being heard, "did you see this month's *Cavemopolitan*? It's the issue on getting in shape! Look at this girl on the cover . . . can you imagine *us* looking like her? If Fred ever happens to see this, his eyes will fall out of his head!" "Wilma, don't be silly," Betty responds, in a rankled tone, "that girl on the cover is sixteen years old and a world-famous model to boot. Besides, if I take off my glasses, close one eye really tight, and squint . . . in very dim light, from a distance, I'd say you look almost as good!"

No matter what your perspective is, there's no denying the truth: In today's world, we're too often judged according to how we look. The proof of this is everywhere and couldn't be any more clear. Whether it's movies, magazines, tabloids, billboards, ads, or shows on TV, we're routinely exposed to images that our society views as "ideal." The message that we're getting from this is disarmingly loud and clear: Doing our best, and being our best, is simply not good enough. What we are failing to see, though, are the facts behind the facade. We don't, for example, when seeing that "perfect" girl on the cover of *Vogue*, give thought to the fact that her sleek, flawless look is usually one that's contrived. Typically, it's an idealized, media-influenced "picture" of health—an image that deftly disguises the fact that the subject *is not* what she seems! The point of making this point is simply that looks can be deceiving. We can't keep letting our ego dictate the way we pursue our goals. It's our ego, in fact, that is often our most formidable UFO.

This chapter examines UFOs that relate to our ego concerns. It reveals how people are often misled by cultural preoccupations and driven to realize standards that are impractical to achieve. It discusses appearance obsession, as well as performance-enhancing drugs, and provides you with valuable insight into the mind-set behind their abuse. In addition, you learn how to screen advice to avoid being led astray.

Withstanding Societal Pressures

When comparing ourselves to a certain ideal is eroding our self-esteem, we're sometimes compelled to take radical steps in an effort to conquer our "flaws." Usually, though, when we do this, the result doesn't please us for long. If we take diet drugs, for example, or if we surgically alter our look, we just feed our starving egos in ways that, at best, provide a quick fix. For each little flaw that we're able to mend (or manage somehow to conceal), we find, over time, once the novelty fades, that a great many more still exist. Being exposed to these images is what's blinding us to the truth—too many of us are pursuing goals that we can't ever hope to achieve. In essence, they're only reflections of our vain, ego-centered world, painted and polished illusions formed to make us buy into a lie! The ultimate irony, though, becomes more clear when considering this: To keep pace with our mythical idols, we're too often *risking our health*. In order to make ourselves look good, we're making ourselves feel bad. We're starving, drugging, and pushing ourselves to potentially harmful extremes.

The following story is true and makes this point especially well. One day, I was at the gym with Jill, a client I'd known for years. Jill, who was in her late twenties, was always in fabulous shape. But although she often was told she looked good, it wasn't quite good enough. Her goal was to make herself perfect, like "those girls in the magazines."

As I listened to her share her feelings about her struggle to lose a few pounds, I felt a great deal of compassion for her and for others who felt the same way. "We don't often do very well," I said, "when we set impractical goals. By comparing ourselves to an image we have of what we consider ideal, we set ourselves up, again and again, to fall disappointingly short. Each time we repeat this pattern, we accrue even more self-doubt. We condition ourselves to *expect* to fail, and we keep on doing just that."

"Sure, that makes perfect sense," said Jill, "but I still can't help how I feel! I mean, just look at that girl over there, the thin one who's wearing the thong. How can I ever compete with that, she's in such phenomenal shape! I'd give anything to be her for a day, just to see what it's like. People like that don't have any idea how it feels to be so insecure."

It was at that moment that Linda, the girl in the thong, started heading our way. "Sorry to interrupt," she said, "but I think I could use your help. Someone suggested I talk to you first, about something I'm planning to do. I'm about to undergo surgery . . . to remove this gross fat from my hips. My appointment is only two days from now, and I'm starting to feel kind of scared. I'm not sure I should be doing this, but the guy that I'm dating insists. He's even threatened to leave me if I don't take this fat off, quick."

Linda broke down and went on to reveal the disastrous state of her life. Besides her eating disorder, addiction to drugs, and low self-esteem, she was in an abusive relationship and about to get fired from her job. Her obsession with diet and exercise kept her away from her family and friends, and she spent almost all her free time by herself, more often than not, at the gym. "It might sound crazy," Linda said, with tears streaming down her face, "but I know if I don't keep working this hard, I'll lose everything I've gained! And despite all the time that it's taken me to get into this kind of shape, I *still* don't look even *anything* like *those girls in the magazines!*"

The pressure we feel to conform, compete, stand out, or measure up has severely warped our perspective of what it means and takes to be fit. Sadly, though, we're oblivious to how much we are being duped. To put this into perspective, imagine yourself doing this: You're assisting a famed photographer who is shooting a beautiful model. You watch as she's primped and painted to enhance her near-perfect face. Her garments are expertly fitted and her hair is elaborately coiffed. The lighting is just about perfect and positioned to hide any flaws. Hundreds of photos are taken, which are then computer enhanced. Now imagine the one that you see is the best of a very large batch. Most likely, it's the one in which she looks least like herself.

Do you think that you're being fair to yourself by comparing yourself to this? Regardless, you probably do it a lot, in ways that you don't even know. If you're male, and you envy the drug-enhanced hulks that are pictured in magazines, or a woman who envies the pencil-thin models depicted in *Glamour* or *Vogue* (or a Victoria's Secret catalog), it's important for you to remind yourself that the image you see *isn't real*. It's more like an artist's rendering in which the model is just a prop. It's one that's been changed and perfected almost as much as a photo can be! At any rate, the big lesson here is something akin to this: Because what you see isn't what you get, you can't really get what you see.

Our self-esteem should not depend on how well we conform to ideals. It should not reflect how skilled we are at changing our appearance. It's not what we see in the mirror that is what should concern us the most. It's the self-respect and self-confidence that we mirror for *others* to see. Although it probably sounds cliché, it's a much undervalued truth: It's the beauty that comes from within that determines how good, over time, we look.

> *Our greatest challenge is to be ourselves in a world that is trying to be like everyone else.*
>
> —RENEE LOCKS

Top Five Ways an Appearance Obsession Creates Common UFOs

1. *It fosters poor eating habits and/or a diet that's overly strict.*
2. *It encourages image disorders and risky cosmetic procedures.*
3. *It fuels exercise addiction.* Training too often or doing too much slows down or inhibits progress and results in higher incidences of injury and/or illness.
4. *Striving to reach impractical goals reinforces feelings of failure.* Frustration, anger, and low self-esteem can trigger rebellious be-

havior and can fuel self-destructive conduct or the decision to stop
working out.

5. *Fickle or desperate thinking leads to impulsive, ill-made decisions*
   (purchasing exercise gimmicks or cheap, ineffective machines, or
   opting for surgical changes that aren't really needed or that pose
   risk).

*Chances of being (or meeting) a woman whose measurements are
36-18-33 (the extrapolated proportions of a Barbie doll): 1 in
100,000.*

—*PLAYBOY* MAGAZINE

◆ EXERCISE ◆

Is an Appearance Obsession Keeping You From Achieving Your Fitness Goals?

Put an X next to each statement that directly applies to you.

—— I'm willing to risk my health (experiment with drugs, have a risky surgical procedure, binge/purge, or use laxatives) to improve my physical appearance.

—— I can't stop buying fitness or image-related magazines.

—— Often my mood depends on how I think I compare to others.

—— I've often had dreams or fantasies of being an actor/actress or model.

—— It takes me more than an hour each day to get showered, dressed, and "fixed up."

—— I think and obsess about losing weight much more than most people I know.

—— I usually put off doing things when I'm heavy or out of shape.

—— When I socialize, or I'm out with friends or a date in a public place, I visit the bathroom numerous times to primp or to "check myself out."

—— More often than not, I judge people according to how they look.

—— I worry that people are judging *me* according to how *I* look.

—— When others tell me I look good, it's seldom the way I feel.

—— I'm a sucker for radical diets, exercise gimmicks, or new fitness fads.

—— I scrutinize photographs of myself and usually see only flaws.

—— I often feel jealous or threatened by those who appear more attractive or fit.

Scoring

1–3: *If you have an appearance fear or concern, it's probably one that is common.* Your problem is likely to play itself out in a very specific way (you overeat at a party when you're jealous of somebody's looks).

4–6: *You're often a little too focused on trying to change the way you look.* Though others may see you as self-assured, attractive, or well-developed, the way you've been able to make yourself look doesn't truly reflect how you feel. If you insist on compromising your health to achieve a particular image, you'll find, over time, that the price you pay is much greater than you expect.

7+: *Your love/hate affair with the mirror is adversely affecting your health.* Unless you begin to address how you feel way down deep, below the surface, your appearance obsession is likely to be a consistent thorn in your side. Be sure to examine the list below of ways to move past this block.

Escaping Appearance Obsession

- *Consider the possibility of a veiled, underlying cause.* These common blocks or disorders can fuel or create an obsession with looks: a low-grade state of depression; an energy block or imbalance; a hidden emotional conflict that contributes to poor self-esteem. If you suspect, as you read this book, that you're plagued by these type of problems, seek out a physician or therapist who is familiar with image disorders. While what you read here may give you a sense of what steps it will help you to take, it's best that you try to address these concerns by seeking professional help.

- *Cut yourself lots of slack.* Don't buy into the hype and the glitz in fashion and health magazines. When you look in the mirror, remind yourself that it's you without pretense or props. When you do feel the urge to compare yourself to a media-driven ideal, pick up this book and do a review of the points that are made in this chapter.

Once you are able to center yourself and reframe your perspective, try to step back and remind yourself that ideals are impractical goals.

◆ *Make a list of your talents, strengths, achievements, and special gifts.* Review the list, reflect on it, and tuck it inside your wallet. Whenever you notice yourself feeling bad about something to do with your looks, make it a point to review the list and add one additional thing (for example, "I'm a kind and considerate person," "I have a beautiful voice," "I own a successful business"). By focusing more on your attributes and the things that you do really well, your state of mind should begin to change, along with your view of yourself. Rather than dwelling on shortcomings, you'll be more aware of your strengths.

◆ *Give yourself a "media break."* Watch less TV, avoid the malls, and put down the magazines. Instead, treat yourself to some quiet time off, away from these common distractions. Remember, each time there's an ad on TV showing someone you view as ideal, you subconsciously pick up the message that, in some way, you don't compare. And if you watch a lot of TV (in excess of three hours a day), you see more than thirty commercials or ads that are apt to evoke this thought. That's 210 per week, or about 11,000 per year! Not to mention the billboards, tabloids, movies, and magazines. A good cure for this kind of brainwash is to go on a three-day "fast." Decide that you will ignore all ads and commercials for three straight days. Doing this periodically helps to flush toxic thoughts from your mind—like denying sun to the unhealthy "seeds" that are sowed by commercials and ads. Avoid being overexposed to them, and they won't be allowed to take root.

Wonder how Hollywood women stay so impossibly slim and fit? Just ask Shannon Tweed, a popular actress and centerfold model: "My daily intake is down to, like, seven sunflower seeds, a cup of soup, half a slice of bread, and a chicken breast. If I stopped, I'd get very, very fat, very, very quickly."

—*TV GUIDE*

Dealing With Other's Egos: How to Expose a Fitness Fraud and Guard Against False Prophets

If you train at a gym, perhaps you remember your very first day as a member. You may have been given some cursory sort of assessment or workout advice. You may even have had a session or two with your very own personal trainer. If you need to have your memory refreshed, it might have gone something like this. "Hi, I'm Vinny, otherwise known as that muscle-bound guy with no neck. Yikes, are you sure that you're up to this? You look like you're ready to croak! Don't worry, though, I've helped plenty of folks who were even worse off than you. We'll start over here on this brand-new machine, the one that takes fat off your tush. Here, try to wedge your flabby white thighs in between these uncomfortable pads. There, I'm sorry it's such a tight fit, but you are, after all, pretty huge, Anyway, use this machine for a while, and soon you might fit through the door. Good, I've shamed you enough for today. Now, you are on your own."

Sometimes you witness the other extreme; you get more help than you need. Some trainers want so much to impress—themselves and everyone else—that they bowl people over with concepts and terms that have most of us scratching our heads. But it's not only just the trainers who, at times, can be full of themselves. It's also the self-proclaimed experts flaunting their wisdom in magazines. Consider the following excerpt from a well-known physique magazine, which in essence compares the hormonal effects of drug use and supplementation:

> *Exercise followed by arginine or glycine administration appears to be a more effectual method of stimulating hGh (somatotropin) secretion from the anterior pituitary gland than by using Sinemet (L-dopa, actually L 3-4 dihydroxyphenylalanine, in combination with carbidopa) which can cause dyskinesis (defective voluntary movement patterns).*

If you're able to understand this, then you must: (a) be a doctor; (b) be a liar; or (c) be frighteningly odd. If your answer is (c), I strongly suggest that you seek professional help. If your answer is (b), I suggest that you stop to reflect on this word of advice: If you can't understand what you read and hear, forget what you read and hear. Or, if you're sort of a masochist, keep trying (and get more confused).

Important Questions to Ask Before You Hire a Personal Trainer

Q: What are your credentials?

Right answer: Here is an updated résumé with a list of my qualifications. You'll see that I have a bachelor's degree in a fitness-related field. You'll also see that I've worked with a whole lot of folks who are just like you. If you need a list of references, I'll be happy to send one your way. And if you have other questions, feel free to call, anytime. Interview other trainers as well, to be sure you find the right fit. You want to make sure that you resonate with their temperament and their beliefs. Consider a trainer's experience, but also rely on your instincts. Knowing that you can trust someone means more than anything else.

Q: How do you motivate clients?

Right answer: Because everyone is so different, there is no one single way. It depends on many variables, like one's goals or one's frame of mind. Sometimes it's based on my instincts and experience working with others. But my primary goal is to help you learn new ways to inspire *yourself.*

Q: Could you say that again in plain English?
Right answer: Yes.

Q: Will you ask me about my health and personal history when we start?

Right answer: Together, we'll do an assessment of your mental and physical health. I'll gather as much information from you as you're willing and able to give. The more *I* know, the more *we'll* know about how we can best proceed.

Q: How long will I have to work with you before I can go on my own?

Right answer: Most people feel very confident after five or six one-hour sessions. Sometimes it's more, sometimes it's less, but we make that decision *together*. It depends, in large part, on your goals, your needs, and current conditioning level, as well as your physical make-up and present state of emotional health.

Top Ten Bits of Advice to Ignore in Your Quest for a Better Body

Follow these guidelines religiously and you're sure to fall short of your goals:

1. *Set lofty, rigid, inflexible goals and pursue them at all costs.* Don't ever cut yourself any slack and be as hard on yourself as you can. Do whatever it takes to succeed, regardless of how much it hurts. Remember, you have to be very strong-willed to commit to a foolish approach, especially if it has harmed you or has never, in fact, really worked.

2. *Hang pictures up on your bedroom wall of the most perfect person you know.* Choose her (or him) as a role model and follow her every move. Eat what she eats, do what she does, and trust everything she says. Forget that you've heard she's been nipped, tucked, and sucked by the world's best cosmetic surgeon. Pretend you don't know that her photos have all been air-brushed and computer-enhanced. These things will only distract you and keep you from staying on track.

3. *If you're failing to make any progress, blame your personal trainer.* If you don't have a personal trainer, use that as your excuse. Whatever the case, blame someone or something other than yourself. By accepting that you're responsible for failing to reach your goals, you'll start feeling badly about yourself, which could lead to low self-esteem. Don't fall into this common trap that will set you up to fail.

4. *Never trust your instincts, even if often they're right*. It makes no sense to trust anything (unless someone says you should). Most people know this instinctively.

5. *Take the word of the "expert" with the biggest and loudest mouth*. Carrying on like a lunatic is the mark of a true professional. Also, trust those who use lots of big words and seem to be fond of jargon. Never mind that you won't understand very much about what they are saying. The more complex their advice is, the more valuable it will be.

6. *Stand naked in front of a mirror and stare at your body's worst flaws*. Observe your protruding abdomen and the unsightly droop of your buttocks. Get a good look at your cellulite and notice the width of your hips. By focusing on these areas, you're sure to become more inspired. Forget all that stuff about loving yourself and accepting yourself as you are. It'll just make you fat and lazy and keep you from staying on course.

7. *Make a decision to go the next step in your quest for a better body*. Starve yourself, try a new drug, or force yourself to throw up. Put on a heavy wool sweater and go for a jog on a hot summer day. Don't make a fuss about feeling sick or like you're about to pass out. It's best if you choose not to let these things prevent you from reaching your goals.

8. *Make sure that you have a partner who is critical of your appearance*. Try to pick one insecure enough to project his self-doubt on you. That way, you'll build up resentment and suppress a whole lot of anger. Anger is often a good thing; it inspires you to push yourself harder. It makes you a lot more determined to meet the goals set for you by your partner. What's good about this is that over time your partner will "raise the bar" higher. So you'll never become complacent; you'll look forward to every new goal.

9. *Make it your prime objective to impress your family and friends*. Forget about getting yourself in shape in order to please yourself—you'd think that by now you'd realize that you probably never will. Being concerned with what others think increases your will to succeed. This is because, despite what you do, most people won't be impressed. In fact, they're apt to ignore you,

especially if they're jealous. This will make you train harder in an effort to get their attention.

10. *Don't buy into that crap about how "everyone makes mistakes."* The people you see who are in the best shape are invariably those who are faultless. If you're not working out like a maniac, or starving yourself like a monk, you'll probably never achieve success and you might as well just give up. Remember: If you're not perfect, you won't be accepted or loved.

Inflating Deflated Egos: How Anabolic Steroids Affect One's Mental and Physical Health

Steroids are potent male hormones that are synthetically reproduced. Taken by many top athletes and physique-conscious folks of both sexes, these drugs, in effect, are a risk-laden means to look huge at the gym or the beach. Taken in varied forms and strengths, steroids function like this: Injected or taken orally, they penetrate muscle cells, attaching to key receptor cites to spur biochemical processes (e.g., protein synthesis). The result is increased strength and muscle mass and a much faster rate of recovery.

As steroids come in a number of forms, their effects will usually vary depending on each individual and the varieties that are combined. If you're privy to some of the gym talk that occurs among those "on the juice," perhaps you're even familiar with some of the better known types of these drugs (for example, Depo-Testosterone, Anadrol, Dianabol, Winstrol, and Deca).

Even though steroids are widely believed to produce some dramatic results, some studies have raised questions regarding the efficacy of their use. I'm one of those who believe, though, that steroids do really work— but perhaps not the way that you've heard that they do, or the way that you've always assumed. If you don't train hard, you don't train right, and if you haven't been blessed with good genes, steroids will never do much for you . . . except maybe make you feel sick. But if you train hard, train right, eat right, and also have muscular genes, they might serve to pump up your ego a bit (and your body a bit as well).

Steroid users are headstrong; they have their defenses down pat.

They're so good at quelling the naysayers that there's rarely much room for debate. Often they say, "I'm taking them under a doctor's supervision. As long as they're properly monitored, steroids pose no risk." It's important to understand, though, that this isn't exactly true. Any drug that *in any way* elicits hormonal changes can never be trusted to work the same way for each different person who takes it. No doctor can know regarding these drugs, in all of their combinations, the short-term or long-term effects that they'll have on each individual person. Moreover, even if *physiologic* responses were always the same, there's still no sure way to predict how these drugs will affect the way someone behaves. For example, users may get depressed or become extremely aggressive, or may suffer from paranoia, delusions of grandeur, or fits of rage. When a person who's using steroids is affected by them in this way, he's apt to ignore the advice he gets, no matter how sound it may be. Furthermore, once he gets used to the way his body has been transformed, he usually finds it difficult to accept being anything less. In this respect, steroids can be a highly addictive drug, so much so that users will often ignore any adverse effects, callously disregarding the ways that these drugs are affecting their health. A physician seldom has much control over someone in this state of mind.

Even if you're fairly certain that you would never use steroids yourself, it's important to be informed about what these drugs can and cannot do. After all, when our workouts fail, we sometimes go to extremes. What drives people to risk their health to achieve such a radical look? Why the obsession to build a physique that has such a subjective appeal? While clearly there is no one answer, the best one I know is this: Steroids thicken the armor that guards a vulnerable, wounded soul. This armor serves as a wall or facade that masks a weak sense of self. But the problem with hiding behind this wall is that someday it has to come down. What people who take these drugs ignore is that someday they'll have to stop.

For those who choose to use steroids, being muscular isn't enough. Their goal is to have a perfect physique to make up for what they lack (self-confidence, self-acceptance). But the irony is that using these drugs just creates even more of a void. Often the bigger and stronger one gets, the harder he is on himself. Once he starts fighting his ego this way, it begs even more to be fed. Then, to suppress his "hunger," he's apt to start taking more drugs. The alternative is for him to accomplish this difficult task by himself, an unlikely choice for a person who's never been satisfied with himself. The allure of achieving perfection becomes an inescapable curse, and to hope to attain what can't be attained is the greatest curse of all.

If you've thought about using steroids, I hope this has changed your mind. Most former users admit that using these drugs was a big mistake. Many have serious fears and concerns about what they have done to their body. Some even fear they'll eventually suffer from latent, long-term effects. If you still have an urge to try these drugs, first do yourself this favor: Seek out those who have used them before and find out how things turned out. It would not be wise to approach anyone who is currently taking these drugs, as he's likely to offer you biased advice that's in rigid defense of his choice. In general, tune into your instincts and always remember to trust your gut: If it doesn't feel like the right thing to do, it's probably best that you don't. One stretch of short-lived glory could mean an entire lifetime of regret.

Pros and Cons of Commonly Used Appearance-Enhancing Drugs

STEROIDS
Pros
- Increased muscle mass and strength
- Less recovery time required between training sessions and sets
- You might finish eighth (instead of fourteenth) in some local physique competition and perhaps get a much taller trophy, or, more praise from your muscle-bound peers.

Cons
- Testicular atrophy (shrunken testicles)
- Cancerous tumors
- Gynecomastia (saggy "breasts")
- Hypertension
- Fluid retention
- Reductions in HDL (the "good" cholesterol)
- Depression
- Uncontrolled emotional outbursts (fits of rage)

◆ Irritability
◆ Marked mood swings
◆ Increased aggression
◆ Insatiable desire for sex
◆ Premature baldness
◆ Rectal bleeding
◆ Dizzy spells
◆ Gallstones
◆ Gastrointestinal disorders
◆ Hepatitis
◆ Severe forms of acne
◆ Cardiac, glandular, and kidney disorders
◆ Visual and auditory delusions
◆ Paranoia
◆ Alopecia (loss of body hair)
◆ Nosebleeds
◆ Tendon/ligament weakness
◆ Jaundice
◆ Prostate enlargement
◆ Decreased sperm count
◆ Impotence (sometimes permanent)
◆ For an indefinite length of time, hormone (testosterone) production slows down (or shuts off) after steroid use stops.

Additional Cons Specific to Women
◆ Enlargement of the larynx (voice box)
◆ Permanent deepening of the voice
◆ Hirsutism (excessive growth of facial and body hair)
◆ Reduced breast size
◆ Enlargement of the clitoris
◆ Uterine atrophy
◆ Irregular menstrual cycles
◆ Ammenorhea (cessation of menstruation)
◆ Increased risk of breast cancer
◆ Increased risk of bearing children with birth defects

HUMAN GROWTH HORMONE (hGh)
Pro
- Studies have shown that hGh can reverse the aging process

Cons
- Enlargement of the jaw and forehead
- A gap between the two front teeth
- Irreversible growth of the extremities
- Sudden death

LAXATIVES
Pro
- Relief of constipation

Cons
- Electrolyte depletion
- Irregular heartbeat
- Stomach cramps
- Nausea
- Vomiting
- Headache

DIURETICS
Pros
- Reduced fluid retention
- Enhanced muscle definition

Cons
- Excessive potassium loss
- Excessive drop in blood pressure (hypotension)
- Dry mouth, excessive thirst
- Blood sugar instability
- Irregular heartbeat
- Adverse drug interactions
- Fatigue

◆ Blurred vision
◆ Dizziness
◆ Mood disturbances
◆ Drowsiness
◆ Weak pulse
◆ Cramps
◆ Weakness

AMPHETAMINES
Pros
◆ Improved alertness and concentration; lengthened attention span
◆ Relief of daytime fatigue (short term)
◆ Increased energy level (short term)

Cons
◆ Irritability
◆ Anxiety
◆ Insomnia
◆ Dry mouth
◆ Rapid heartbeat
◆ Hyperactivity
◆ High fever
◆ Hallucinations
◆ Suicidal/homicidal tendencies
◆ Convulsions
◆ Coma
◆ Mood disturbances
◆ Appetite loss
◆ Stomach cramps
◆ Nausea
◆ Chest pain
◆ Involuntary movements of head, neck, arms, and legs
◆ Impotence
◆ Adverse drug interactions
◆ Addiction
◆ Rash, hives

PART II

Keys to Overcoming Mind/Body UFOs*

◆ ◆ ◆

(*Unidentified Fitness Obstacles)

Psychological UFOs

Overcoming Emotional Blocks to Lifelong Physical Fitness

One often meets his destiny on the road he takes to avoid it.

—French proverb

As most of us struggle to get into shape, we focus on fixing our body. Too often, though, we fail to address our feelings regarding the process. Why don't we have time to exercise? Why aren't we more inspired? Why can't we be more disciplined? These are some of the questions that are answered in this chapter.

This chapter reveals emotional blocks that can keep you from getting fit. By examining common UFOs that stem from your negative thoughts, you'll see how, more than you realize, your body believes what you think. In addition, you'll see how perfectionism, depression, and image disorders are all very common UFOs that too often go overlooked. You'll learn how to keep these UFOs, and others, from acting as blocks.

Repressed Anger/Passive Aggression

June has been struggling for more than a year to lose a few extra pounds. Her husband, Ward, hasn't been much help; in fact, he's a thorn in her side. "Off to the gym today, honey?" he inquires in a hopeful tone. "Of course," she snaps, "why do you ask, and why do you seem so concerned?" "Well, in this month's *Playboy*," Ward replies, "there's this babe on page twenty-four. . . ."

June promptly turns her back to him and slams the door in his face. "Honey, what's wrong?" Ward asks, concerned, as he jiggles the lock on the door. "Nothing, I'm fine, just leave me alone," June mutters, while drying her tears. "Why did I have to marry such an insensitive, chauvinist jerk? Why can't you be more like Eddie . . . you know, that well-mannered friend of the Beav?"

From this point on, June claims that she's "too busy" to go to the gym. She observes that her clothes are a bit more snug and she starts feeling more depressed. "What's the use?" she says to herself. "I'm fighting a losing cause. I'll never compare to those centerfold girls, no matter how hard I try. . . ."

If part of this story is ringing a bell, it will help you to keep this in mind: If the reason you're trying to get in shape is to pacify someone else, you're bound to struggle to reach your goals and will, in all likelihood, fail. Why? Because as you start building resentment, trying to look like someone's ideal, you start to repress your anger in ways that prevent you from getting in shape. How can your pent-up feelings act as a block to improving your health? Often, unexpressed anger triggers a passive-aggressive response. When this occurs, you exact revenge by acting out hidden rage. For example, you might "forget" to work out or begin to neglect your appearance, or perhaps even feign an injury, or decide to go on a binge. This unconscious "I'll show you" response is more common than you might expect. Usually, those who react this way aren't even aware that they do. Their old, self-defeating reflexes are triggered by subconscious thoughts.

If you fail to express your anger, it eventually makes itself heard. You can't just deny your feelings, hoping that someday they'll go away. You have to express to others what you most want for yourself. When you share your pain, express your fears, and admit to the ways you feel wounded, your loved ones can see the impact of their demands and expectations. You must set and enforce healthy boundaries and learn to have more self-respect. Once people know that you won't be abused, they stop rubbing salt in your wounds.

It's important that others are crystal clear about how to support you best. It is your task to enlighten them, to tell them what will (and won't) help. What can be done to make you feel more positive and inspired? Would it help if your partner was building you up instead of breaking you down—doing his best to applaud your success instead of exposing your flaws? Don't assume that he or she knows that this is the right thing to do. You've already had enough evidence to confirm that this isn't the case.

Building and Breaking Down Walls: Coming to Terms with a History of Physical/Mental Abuse

To experience personal growth, we must expose and face our fears. We often forget how our fears keep us from doing what serves us best.

Those who have suffered abuse, for example, rebel against getting in shape, when the message that keeps playing back to them is that "looking *too* good is *bad*." For them, the notion of getting in shape taps into a deep-seated fear. Although they may *say* they want to lose weight, and *appear* to be battling their bulge, they may really be staging an inward fight with a fear of feeling unsafe. Their weight may serve as a safeguard or as a physical shield for their soul, dissuading those who, if not "walled out," might attempt to find a way in. But although this wall may insulate them from those they perceive as a threat, it may also keep them from getting in touch with the way they really feel. In this respect, although this shield may help keep people away, it may also serve as a barrier to connecting with one's own truth. The longer that you deny yourself and ignore what you know in your heart, the less you'll be able to move past your fears, and the thicker your wall will become.

How can you take down this wall? If you've had any history of abuse, regardless of how it occurred, I'm not going to kid you by making it sound like it will be an effortless task. In fact, I very strongly suggest that you seek some professional help. Here, the intent is merely to show how the "wall" can be linked to your fears, to awaken you to the notion that, perhaps, it's what's holding you back.

We often suppress or deny those fears that are hardest for us to face. It's possible that the depth of your pain runs deeper than you even know, so deep, in fact, that you have little faith that this pain can be overcome. But it can, and it will, if you're open enough to express how you *really* feel. You need ongoing support, though, to achieve ongoing growth. Without it, the wall that you've built for yourself may be simply too hard to tear down.

> *I didn't know that hurt goes away faster if one is willing to feel it, perhaps shed some tears, and let it pass, instead of spending huge amounts of energy denying it. I'm learning that I can say no and watch a relationship deepen instead of disappear. I'm learning that I can like myself, even though I'm not perfect. I'm learning that letting down my guard and telling it like it is brings others closer rather than pushing them away.*
>
> —ELIZABETH

How Family and Friends Can Influence How You Feel About Getting Fit: Rising Above "Boundary Bashers" and Your Old, Disempowering Beliefs

"Ellie May, where have you been?" Granny screeched. "Your lunch has been ready since noon. The least you could do is git here on time—you know how I hate when you're late! Look, I fixed you your favorite, Kentucky-fried possum an' grits! C'mon, set down, you need to eat before these here vittles git cold!"

"Why heck, Granny, I ain't late," Ellie said. "It ain't even close to noon! And why did ya' have to go fixin' all this foul-smellin', vein-cloggin' food? How many times have I told ya' that I'm fixin' to lose some weight? How did ya' reckon I'd ever be able to eat all this fatnin' grub? Heck, I ain't no Jethro, you know. I'd barf if I chowed all this slop!"

"Dad blast it, Ellie," Granny growled, "don't tell me you ain't gonna eat!? Imagine, I slaved all night and all day, an' this is the thanks I git! Why are you dieting, anyway? You're startin' to look like a twig! Even your Uncle Jed's been concerned; he thinks your face looks too thin. Here, set down an' eat somethin', child. You need to put meat on dem bones!"

Whether it's how they act, choose words, or use the tone of their voice, the way that your family relates to you can affect how you view getting fit. For example, some parents are skilled at provoking guilt as a means of control, often to keep family members tied to traditional roles or events. If you can relate, and you're feeling some guilt about getting yourself into shape, perhaps it's time to consider the role that your parents and siblings have played. In Ellie's case, it was Granny who starred in the guilt-generating role. Her act was performed to discourage Ellie's resolve to lose any more weight. If you, too, are being undermined by your relatives, family, or friends, it might be a good idea for you to start putting them in their place. In the end, you'll really be serving them best by taking good care of yourself.

Your family may also influence how you feel about how you look. For example, if most of your family could, in a word, be described as "stout," you might be afraid, because of your genes, that you'll suffer a similar fate. This may cause you to view yourself with a keen, hypercritical eye. As your family watches you do this, they may start becoming unnerved. They may be concerned that you'll be judging *them* based on standards you've set for yourself. Thus, they may try to dissuade you from pursuing your fitness goals. Whatever the case, when this occurs, you'll be challenged to stay on course. If your family keeps making it hard for you to persist as you strive to get fit, it's unlikely if this continues that your path will lead to success.

Sometimes, it's friends and acquaintances who attempt to lead you astray. For example, let's say you've lost twenty-five pounds and you're pleased with the way you look. So you purchase a sexy, form-fitting dress to wear to a holiday party. Imagine you're at the party and you run into one of your friends. "The time you looked your best," she says, "was last year at Julie's party. I know you said you were ill that day and had put on a whole lot of weight, but I must say, you did look more youthful wearing that baggy, conservative dress."

Or let's say you're a man whose primary goal is to look more defined. Imagine that you've lost ten pounds of fat and gained several pounds of muscle. But your buddy, whom you haven't seen for a while, isn't comfortable with the new you. "Took some time off from the gym," he asks, "or have you been slacking off? Wow, take a look in the mirror. Next to me, you look really small. You better start hitting the iron again, or people will think something's wrong!"

In both of these cases, the saboteurs felt threatened and insecure.

Their comments reflected how poorly they felt about how they believed they compared. If you can relate, it's important that you learn to see this for what it is. If you take the bait, get mad at your friends, and begin to question yourself, you'll just have to live with your low self-esteem while *they* live rent free in your head. So your best options are to "evict" them, or to insist that they "pay you rent" (in other words, tell you honestly exactly the way that they feel). Either way, it's better than putting up with their hurtful remarks. Determining what lies beneath them is the best way to make them stop.

Dealing with "Boundary Bashers"

SET AND ENFORCE HEALTHY BOUNDARIES

Tell family members, coworkers, and friends that you'd like to enlist their help. Tell them how much it would mean to you to have their consistent support as you make a commitment to exercise more, lose weight, or improve your health. Explain to them how important it is for you to accomplish your goals, and that if they'd like to support you, you'd prefer only "pats on the back" (for example, "You're doing great," "Keep up the good work," "I can see that it's paying off"). If they keep saying things that are hurtful or in some way are out of line, insist in a firm but dispassionate way that they keep their critiques to themselves. If you can't imagine a tactful way to make this kind of request, you might want to try what a friend of mine does (or something along the same lines). Whenever she's being criticized, or someone just won't shut up, she crosses her eyes, plugs up her ears, and whistles a sprightly tune. I've been at the other end of this, and I have to admit that it works. It works because it makes her point in a lighter, less pointed way.

Another option is making your critics explain what's behind their remarks. You might hear them say, for example, "I fear that you're judging the way that *I* look." Or, "I have to admit that, at times, I'm envious of your success." You might be surprised by how well most people respond to this kind of request. Often they welcome the chance to express the way that they truly feel.

USE THE IMAGO DIALOGUE PROCESS

When your efforts to eat right and exercise are rebuked by your family and friends, you may feel a need to stand up for yourself, or to get them to see things your way. But whenever you act defensively or try to argue your point, what usually ends up happening is that your feelings don't get heard.

One great way to help others to be more attuned to the way you feel is by using the Imago dialogue process, created by Harville Hendrix. In essence, it works like this: First, approach the person with whom you have a specific concern. Then, ask if he or she's willing to give you a chance to share how you feel. The key to making this process work is abiding by this simple rule: Each person must only *mirror*, or reflect, what the other says. So instead of getting defensive and reacting to things that are said, you simply repeat whatever you hear in a flat, nonjudgmental way. By starting with certain key phrases that will help guide your feelings and thoughts (*I think, I feel, I imagine, I hope, I worry*, etc.), you begin to uncover the truth about some of your feelings, fears, and concerns. If you start, for example, by saying, "I think that you envy the way that I look," your partner says, very simply, "You think that I envy the way that you look." Your partner does not say, "You're crazy," "You're out of your mind," or "You're full of crap." Instead, he or she just repeats what you say, without an interpretation.

The beauty of this is that mirroring (rather than being defensive or mad) enables a level of empathy that is rarely achieved other ways. As the process unfolds, and you both have a chance to be heard as you share how you feel, your defenses break down, you start to build trust, and you start to see things a new way. You find that once people start hearing you, you're open to hearing them too.

Depression: Common Effects on Physical Health and Physical Fitness Potential

Kathy: I think I've done all that I possibly can to get into better shape. Nothing seems to work for me, though. I must be a hopeless case. I'm still overweight, I hate how I look, and I couldn't be more depressed. If only I were a lot thinner, then, my whole life would change!

Michael: Kathy, can you remember a time when you liked the way you looked?

Kathy: Sure, back when I was in high school. Of course, I weighed twenty pounds less.

Michael: So then you were a lot happier . . . ?

Kathy: I guess, now that I look back on it, I felt much like I do now. I've always been pretty hard on myself, even when I was a kid.

Michael: How long have you been unhappy? Was there a time that you weren't depressed?

Kathy: I don't think I'm *depressed*, like *sick*, if that's what you mean to suggest. Besides, I go to work every day, I even laugh once in a while. There's no way that I could be really depressed. If I were, I'd be sad all the time!

Michael: Regarding your view of depression, it's not about what you *can* do, it's more about what you *can't*. When you're feeling depressed, for example, is it harder for you to lose weight? As a trainer, I've found that depression can actually act as a physical block. It can sometimes affect your body even more than it does your mind. What has kept you from fully accepting yourself and deriving much joy from your life may actually be the very same thing that has kept you from getting in shape. While a low-grade state of depression may not *prevent* you from living your life, it could *limit* you in some critical ways that will keep you from living it well.

Like many, you may look at getting in shape as a cure for a long list of ills. You might even think that by reaching your goals, you wouldn't feel so depressed. But perhaps it's not falling short of your goals that is making you feel depressed. Perhaps, instead, it's because you're depressed that you've been falling short of your goals. When I think about all of the clients I've had with a history of low-grade depression, it's hard to believe that so few of them had any sense it was holding them back. It's hard to believe that despite how they felt, so few of them sought any help! But then I try to remind myself what it's like to be truly depressed: You blame yourself, you deny your thoughts, and you doubt that your mood will improve. In addition, you doubt that the actions you take will produce a successful result (for example, "Why bother to exercise? I know that I'll always be fat"). Add in the stigma that's often attached to admitting that you're depressed, and it's no wonder so few admit to themselves, or to others, the way they feel. Unless people face the truth, though, they continue to spin their wheels, whether they're struggling to better their life or struggling to better their health.

If you *are* depressed, and you're worried it means that there's something incredibly wrong, imagine instead that it means your emotions have simply become flattened out. It simply means that your "engine" (your mind) in effect needs some tuning up. It doesn't mean that you're sick, or weak, or a hopeless, pathetic mess. Nor does it mean that big men in white coats will be hot on your trail, waving nets. What it does mean, though, is that if your depression has lasted a fairly long time (more *often* than not, more *days* than not, and also for more than *three months*), you should see an experienced therapist who can help you to get back on track—at the very least, to assure yourself that you're not clinically depressed. But if you are, don't worry. In fact, you happen to be in luck. The good news about depression is that with treatment, you can be helped.

◆ EXERCISE ◆

Is a Low-Grade State of Depression Expressing Itself as a UFO?

Put an X next to each statement that relates to the way you feel.

—— It's hard for me to stay focused on how it might help me to get into shape. Instead, I think about how I might feel if I don't force myself to work out (for example, "My health will suffer," "I won't look as good as my friends").

—— I don't believe that I have what it takes to get myself into shape. I don't have the patience or fortitude to keep myself on the right path.

—— I often crave sugary, fat-laden foods when I'm bored or in a bad mood.

—— I don't acknowledge compliments. I don't believe they're deserved.

—— When I think about how I've struggled to lose weight and to get into shape, I usually start to get down on myself and assume that it's all my fault.

—— I often feel apathetic, like nothing I do really counts.

—— I can't imagine in any way feeling good when I work out.

—— Unlike what I hear is often the case, working out doesn't help my mood.

—— I'm very sensitive to criticism, particularly about my appearance.

—— Working out feels like too much of a chore. It's not worth the effort it takes.

—— When I do work out, more often than not I move at a leisurely pace, like something is "weighing me down" or making me sluggish, lethargic, and slow.

—— Compared to others my size and age, I can't handle physical stress. I don't seem to have much tolerance. When I train, I'm often in pain.

—— I've lost (or gained) a whole lot of weight (more than 5 percent of my body weight) all in the course of one month.

—— More often than not, I sleep too much (or I don't get enough *good* sleep).

—— I often feel very guilty about taking the time to work out.

—— I have a hard time staying focused, even on simple, everyday tasks.

Scoring

1–3: *You're probably being affected by some other UFO.* By addressing additional UFOs that are strictly related to you, any depressive symptoms you have should eventually start to subside.

4–6: *It's possible that you're suffering from a low-grade state of depression (dysthymia).* This can be a tough call, though, if your symptoms are varied or vague. In addition, when symptoms of UFOs are similar or overlap, you need to find out if it's possible that they are rooted in some other problem (for example, some type of allergy or a problem related to sleep). If, in general, your mood seems mostly okay, and you do attempt to work out, you may find that if you can do it enough, exercise actually helps. But the paradox with depression is that although working out *can* help, those who are more than just mildly depressed *may not have the will to persist.* If this is also the case for you, your efforts may well be in vain—unless you take steps to address how you feel *before* you make plans to work out.

7–9: *There's a very good chance that you're suffering from a chronic form of depression.* Again, you should see a professional to expose the specific cause. If you fail to address your depression, working out isn't likely to help, mostly because when your efforts are forced, you set yourself up to fail. In short, if your fuel tank is leaking, and you force yourself to work out, before long your engine will sputter and you'll find yourself out of gas. Instead of believing that pushing yourself is the only real option you have, address how you feel and enlist some support to help get yourself back on track.

10+: *You probably won't learn much from this test that you haven't already suspected.* But sometimes, assessing yourself in this way can incite you to take some action. The sooner that you receive qualified help, the sooner you'll start feeling better. Ask someone you trust to assist you in making the right connection, or turn to the Appendix to find the right professional help.

◆ ◆ ◆

Depression is merely anger, without enthusiasm.
—STEVEN WRIGHT

Symptoms of Major Depression

At least five of the following:

- Depressed mood
- Diminished interest or pleasure in all, or almost all, activities
- Significant weight gain or weight loss (5 percent or more in a month)
- Insomnia or hypersomnia nearly every night
- Restlessness or lethargy noted by others most every day
- Fatigue or loss of energy nearly every day
- Feelings of worthlessness or extreme guilt

- Dulled thinking, difficulty concentrating
- Recurrent thoughts of dying or suicide

Symptoms of Long-Term, Low-Grade Depression (Dysthymia)

Depressed or irritable mood (for most of the day, more days than not, and for at least two years) AND at least two of the following:

- Poor appetite or overeating
- Insomnia or hypersomnia
- Low energy or fatigue
- Low self-esteem
- Poor concentration or difficulty making decisions
- Feelings of hopelessness

So what ever happened to Kathy, once we revealed that she was depressed? After some counseling sessions, in which we exposed and addressed her fears, Kathy observed that, in general, she was feeling more self-assured. But although she did make some headway and felt more secure overall, a check to determine her status revealed that there wasn't much change in her mood. She then went to see a psychiatrist, who confirmed that she still was depressed. After only six weeks of treatment (with an antidepressant drug), she said that it somehow had strengthened her and helped her to "reclaim her soul." She couldn't believe how different she felt—and how different she *looked*. The things that once were so hard for her all of a sudden weren't hard at all. She lost fifteen pounds, stepped up her routine, and began to enjoy working out. But the best part of it all was that she learned to accept herself. She was happy to do the best that she could, regardless of what she achieved.

It's important to note that even though Kathy's condition was helped with a drug, this treatment approach may not necessarily be what is best for you. A change in your diet (or counseling) may be all that you really need. If you're like Kathy, though, and the use of a drug is appropriate in your case, you should know that if it's prescribed the *right way*, there's only a *minimal* risk. It's too bad that there's such a stigma attached to antidepressant drugs, because it keeps us from celebrating the fact that they save and enhance people's lives. Until I was able to see for myself how these drugs helped a lot of my clients, my feeling was that, for the most part, they were too often used as a crutch. I also believed that these drugs just masked, or covered up, difficult feelings, and that people who took them were lazy, weak, or taking the easy way out. Now I believe that these drugs give people the strength to *confront* their feelings, and that sometimes some people need these drugs to reset a blown "mental fuse." I've seen too many people transform their lives after using these drugs a short time to pretend that long-term psychotherapy is a smarter or nobler choice.

If it seems a bit strange that I advocate drugs in a book with a mind/body bent, it's because I feel that a holistic cure shouldn't preclude the *sound* use of meds. Sometimes, all things considered, it's simply what makes the most sense. If a mood disturbance is rooted in some type of biochemical imbalance, it's unlikely that simply "talking it out" will go a long way to help. This is akin to discussing the cause of a rapidly sinking ship, which is okay to do if the ship isn't actually sinking, *while you're aboard*. Once you know that the hole is there, and the water is filling your boat, it must be patched well before you consider your thoughts about how it occurred. In this sense, these drugs are a lifesaver; they won't allow you to drown. They'll help keep your head above water so you can see your way clear to the shore.

In spite of increasing awareness regarding medical help for depression, most people still perceive mood-changing drugs as an option that poses some risk, especially ever since Fen-Phen (Fenfluramine and Phentermine) was revealed to have caused some harm (i.e., heart-valve damage). But Fen-Phen, unlike other drugs that have safely been used for years, was never extensively studied or put to a valid, long-term test. In addition, antidepressant drugs affect people different ways. A drug that works very well for one, may not work so well for another. And although drugs like Prozac and Paxil are *at times* linked to adverse effects, on the whole the negative media reports have been vastly overblown. For every one person who's taken these drugs and has had a particular problem, there're hundreds, perhaps even thousands of folks, who have not and who've found that they've helped.

It's important for you to bear in mind that antidepressants *are* safe, as long as they're taken properly and have passed a long-term test. Moreover, the way that these drugs are fine-tuned can vary from doctor to doctor, so it helps to find one who's committed to finding precisely what works for you best. A sensitive doctor prescribes these drugs *only* when they are needed, and then ensures when you take them that they're not causing you any harm. He or she should also be aware of your family history, in addition to how your personal needs (biochemically) are unique. Drug interactions and side effects should also be considered, as well as alternative options, like St. John's Wort and bright lights. Some doctors do prescribe these drugs in a careless or casual manner, so be sure, if you do choose to take them, that you've made a well-informed choice.

It may also be that, like Kathy, your treatment will be short term, used in large part as a springboard simply to help you get back on track. When Kathy completed her treatment, not once did she ever look back. She's been happy and healthy ever since and has never regretted her choice.

If you are suffering from depression, once the problem has been resolved, you'll see a dramatic, positive shift in your energy level and mood. Things that at one time were tedious, like dieting or working out, will suddenly feel like a challenge that you're ready to meet head-on. Instead of dwelling on how life will be if you *don't* get yourself into shape, you'll start thinking more about how it will be once you're feeling more healthy and fit. You'll feel like a whole different person—and in time, you'll look like one too.

Not everything that is faced can be changed, but nothing can be changed until it is faced.

—JAMES BALDWIN

Top Ten Ways to Overcome a Low-Grade State of Depression

1. *Responsible use of the right kind of drug, prescribed by a skilled physician.*

2. *Acupuncture, acupressure, or electro-acupuncture.* Electro-acupuncture has proved to be an effective option (refer to the Appendix for additional information).

3. *St. John's Wort* (not to be used in combination with other antidepressants, except for in certain instances, when prescribed by a skilled physician).

4. *Thought-field therapy (TFT).*

5. *Nutritional modification* (with attention to food combinations, food allergies, food intolerances, and insulin sensitivity).

6. *Overcoming addictions* (for example, alcohol, caffeine, or tobacco). See additional information regarding TFT.

7. *Adjusting to seasonal changes* (winter blues or SAD).

8. *Addressing hormonal changes* (PMS, menopause, postpartum depression).

9. *Counseling/psychotherapy* (addressing suppressed emotions, in particular, anger and rage).

10. *Staying connected with others* (building a solid support network, developing long-term friendships).

Perfectionism: How It Fuels Fitness Failure

Donna was a perfectionist who was obsessed with doing her best. No matter what project or task she took on, she always gave it her all. Her objective was plain and simple: never to make a mistake. "If I do," she said, "I'm afraid, someday, the world might discover the truth—that underneath this perfect mask I'm really a perfect fraud."

Donna had always been hard on herself and often downplayed her success. But her parents were hard on her also, as they felt she had underachieved. They had set high standards for Donna and had pressured her to excel. "There's no mountain," Donna's dad told her, "that is too high for you to climb." Sadly, though, she was seldom praised or acknowledged for what she achieved. Her parents feared that by doing so, they'd encourage her to be lax. They worried that she would "get a big head" and be less inspired to succeed.

While Donna did find a way to accomplish most of her lofty goals, she consistently found herself struggling when it came to improving her health. Despite the fact that she ate well and worked out at least six days a week, Donna could not break a habit that flew in the face of her perfect act. She'd been smoking two packs of cigarettes, every day, for about ten years.

"I started when I was eighteen," Donna said, "while living alone at school. Being away from my parents was both a blessing and a curse. On one hand, I felt like a lab rat that had escaped from my parents' cage. I enjoyed my new-found freedom and I liked being out on my own. But my parents feared that I might slack off if they weren't always on my case. So although I had begged them not to, they called me at least *twice a day*. They usually asked lots of questions and wanted reports on my latest grades. Meanwhile, I was struggling to keep my 4.0 average intact. I recall at the time being really upset by the way my parents behaved. That's when I started smoking, I think as a way to rebel. I guess what I liked most about it was escaping my good girl role. It was like I was making a statement, kind of like, 'Mom and Dad, this butt's for you!' To this day, when I'm feeling angry or pressured to do perfect work, I find that it's almost impossible to control my urge to smoke. It feels like this weird kind of reflex that I don't have the power to stop!"

Instead of relaxing her standards, or confronting her mom and dad, Donna's response to "perfectionist stress" was to reach for a cigarette. Smoking, to her, was a reflex that was mainly set off by two things: the pressure that she would put on herself, and the pressure she got from her parents. Once Donna made this connection, she could see how it all played out. More and more, as time went on, whenever she craved a smoke, she slowed herself down, took a deep breath, and thought about *why* she did. And when her parents pressured her or meddled in her affairs, she gently but firmly insisted they stop and keep their beliefs to themselves.

Did Donna stop having cravings once she began to confront her parents? Although she made some progress, there was still more work to be done. Her cravings *did* stop completely once her energy blocks were released. The way that Donna accomplished this was through treatment with thought-field therapy (see Chapter 1). We found that she was reversed around the issue of being perfect. She also had a block related to self-acceptance and trust. The energy in her body that existed around these issues was blocked in a way that intensified her compulsive urge to smoke. Once we peeled back the layers, and treated them one by one, Donna was well on her way to living a healthier, smoke-free life. She started to find that by doing less, she achieved a great deal more.

◆ **EXERCISE** ◆

Are You Trying to Be Too Perfect?
Has Perfectionistic Behavior Been
at the Root of Your Fitness Failure?

Put an X next to each statement that directly applies to you:

——— My attitude about exercise is that it has to be all or none. If I can't do the "perfect" workout, I won't exercise at all.

——— I procrastinate. My need to do everything flawlessly makes me put off important tasks (for example, getting myself to the gym or changing the way I eat).

——— It's hard for me to trust advice or to ask anyone for help.

——— I worry about feeling pressured, being judged, or being controlled.

——— I'm usually very sensitive to comments about how I look.

——— I tend to avoid the gym when I don't believe I look my best.

——— When working out, I wear loose clothes to hide what I think are my flaws.

——— If I happen to miss a workout, I feel a great deal of guilt. It's usually very hard for me to rest or take time off.

——— I find it hard to trust that things will really turn out for the best.

——— I easily get embarrassed if I'm being admired or praised.

——— I'm my own worst critic. It's hard to accept myself.

——— I tend to be superstitious about how I train and what I eat. I feel depressed or unsettled if I do something different or wrong.

——— I keep meticulous records. I need to write everything down in order to feel like I'm in control.

—— I often work so long or hard in pursuit of professional goals that I seldom have time for exercise, let alone much of anything else. Taking the time to exercise seems like it's not a "responsible" choice.

—— It's hard for me to deviate very much from my normal routine.

Scoring

1–2: *It's unlikely that perfectionism is the root cause of your problem.* The ways you tend to be hard on yourself may relate more to other blocks.

3–5: *Your perfectionistic tendencies are undoubtedly slowing your progress.* To understand how this can occur, review the list below.

6+: *With regard to physical fitness, you're trying to be "too perfect."* Too perfect means that as hard as you try, you'll *never* achieve your goals. It's time to come to terms with the truth and to curb your perfectionist bent. You'll find that once you start doing so, your workouts will start working out.

◆ ◆ ◆

Three Ways to Keep Perfectionism from Being a UFO

1. *Contact a thought-field therapist.* Perfectionism is often linked to energy blocks in the body. Conventional forms of counseling can help free up some of these blocks, but if they run deep, or are numerous, you may want to try TFT (see Appendix for references).

2. *Wake up to the realization that you're setting unreachable goals.* Instead of always obsessing about the goals you've failed to achieve, make it a point each day to review the things that you've done really well. Before setting goals, always ask yourself if they're truly within your grasp. Then ask yourself if they're practical, given what it would take to succeed. If instead of seeking perfection, "excellence" is your goal, you'll find yourself feeling more centered, more self-aware, and more self-assured. By learning to frame it this way, you at least have a chance to succeed.

3. *Find out if your need to be perfect stems from additional UFOs.* As you read this book, consider how other obstacles could be

involved. If you have ADD (attention deficit disorder), for example, and it's hard for you to stay focused, you may feel you have to be perfect in order to compensate for this "flaw." Once you have finished reading this book, and you're able to see the whole picture, you shouldn't have trouble determining which UFOs should be dealt with first.

How an Addiction to Exercise Can Be a UFO

Hello, my name is Michael, and I am an exercise addict. There, I said it, admitted the truth, got it right off my chest. Currently, though, I'm arguably much less obsessed than I've ever been, which basically means that although I do less, I probably still do too much. But at least I can say that I'm much better now than I was at drawing the line. For example, if I had mono right now, I wouldn't keep working out (believe it or not, several years ago this was something I actually did). But the thing that I still find surprising, now that I don't work out quite as much, is not just that I feel better, but that I'm actually in better shape. I'm leaner, stronger, and healthier than I was when I did a lot more. It's taken me years to accept this, but I now know that less *is* more.

What makes an exercise addict? Most people I know who are, or were, addicted to working out are those with a long-storied history of feeling a need to be in control—particularly of their body—based on traumatic events in their past. Some examples are being an overweight youth who was teased by his or her peers, or someone who's seen a relative suffer with poor or failing health. Most addicts also have low self-esteem, though they hide this amazingly well. Much of what tends to fuel them is a fear that they're actually frauds, a fear that they'll look bad or average if they don't push themselves to extremes. Exercise addicts also contend that they're "different" from everyone else, that they feel compelled to work harder than most to experience any success. In addition, they usually fit into one of the following classifications.

Variations of Exercise Addicts

◆ *Narcissists.* Narcissists cannot separate who they are from the way they look. They try to perfect their bodies to fulfill their need for praise.

◆ *Perfectionists.* Perfectionists seldom are confident that they've ever worked out enough. They believe that by training excessively and/ or forcing themselves to do more, they'll succeed in making up for the ways they feel vulnerable, lacking, or weak. They tend to think, "If there is no pain, there won't be significant gain."

◆ *Anorexics, bulimics, or those who suffer with other image disorders.* Some people's warped self-perceptions cause them to do self-destructive things. While they often go to harmful extremes to alter the way they look, their problem is how they *think and feel* as opposed to how they appear. The measures they take to make themselves "right" are exactly what makes them go wrong.

◆ *Avoidance personalities.* Some people overexercise to escape from the trials of their life. Working out is an excuse they use to avoid facing difficult things.

◆ *Obsessive-compulsives.* Compulsive exercisers need a precisely structured routine. They fret about minute details and often push themselves to extremes. Even when they are injured, weak from fatigue, or feeling ill, they refuse to slow down or to take time off, for fear that they'll lose what they've gained.

Top Ten Ways an Addiction to Exercise Can Be a UFO

1. *An exercise addiction causes compulsive overtraining.*

2. *Exercise addicts suffer from greater workout-related stress.* Exercise addicts tend to obsess about details involving their training, such as doing enough, doing what's best, or not having adequate time.

3. *An exercise addiction leads to self-destructive practices* (crash diets, overexertion, and training when injured or ill).

4. *Sufficient time is not allowed for peak recovery and growth*. Because those addicted to exercise frequently train several times a day, rest phases between workouts are often too short to enable gains.

5. *Exercise addicts often refuse to take periodic breaks*. Occasional layoffs are needed to renew one's body and soul.

6. *Exercise addicts often exclude activities that provide balance* (social activities and fun forms of recreation). A narrow focus on fitness can often result in these UFOs: depression, chronic fatigue, anxiety, depression, sleep problems, body image/eating disorders, and obsessive/compulsive tendencies.

7. *The "plateau phases" addicts experience are more frequent and more prolonged* (periods during which progress slows or grinds to a sudden halt).

8. *An addiction to exercise often creates or exacerbates energy blocks* (self-defeating thoughts, or feeling stuck, lethargic, or stale).

9. *A long-term addiction to exercise can lead to a state of reversal, a "polarized," counterproductive belief that prevents the achievement of goals*. (Psychological reversal is discussed in Chapter 1.)

10. *Exercise addicts typically make inefficient use of their time*. Training too long or too often is likely to slow or restrict one's progress.

◆ EXERCISE ◆

Are You an Exercise Addict?

Put an X next to each statement that directly applies to you.

—— I feel very anxious whenever I think about *missing* my normal routine.

—— I feel very anxious whenever I think about *changing* the way I work out.

—— I must keep a rigid schedule. I resist taking any time off.

—— I'm often compelled to complete the specific routine that I have planned,

—— regardless of injury, illness, or extenuating factors (bad weather, obligations, or unexpected events).

—— I'm superstitious about what I do and about how often I do it (for example, ''I have to train every day. If I don't, my muscles will shrink'').

—— I feel anxious, depressed, and irritable if I can't do my normal routine.

—— When I work out, I feel anxious if I feel that I'm pressured for time.

—— After completing a workout, I feel a great deal of relief.

—— Before I begin a workout, I feel a great deal of stress.

Scoring

At least 4: Moderate workout addiction.

5+: Significant workout addiction. Consider the following suggestions to conquer this UFO.

◆ ◆ ◆

Four Keys to Overcoming an Exercise Addiction

1. *Identify and address your other related UFOs.* It's possible, even likely, that there are other blocks involved (for example, depression, low self-esteem, perfection, or energy blocks). By uncovering those that are hindering you most, you'll see how they fuel your addiction. Then, once you start to address them, your addiction will loosen its hold. Behavior that once was a reflex for you will no longer seem to make sense. You'll find yourself feeling more clear about what kinds of actions serve you best.

2. *Thought-field therapy.* An addiction to exercise often has roots in emotional problems or fears (low self-esteem, body image disorders, a fear of criticism, or perfectionism). Blocks around these issues respond very well to TFT.

3. *Consider a brief trial period during which you exercise less.* If you try a routine that is shorter as well as less strenuous than the norm, you can see for yourself if it really does help you more to be doing less. If you track your results objectively and make notes about how you feel, you should actually find that

in most ways your fitness level *improves*. As soon as you have some proof of this, you may start to feel less obsessed. Always remember this critical point that is too often overlooked: The key to success isn't how *much* you do, it's how you *do* what you do.

4. *Reframe your perspective. Focus on training efficiently as opposed to doing too much.* If you exercise hard, your workouts are brief, and your efforts are safe and sound, you're doing everything possible to ensure your greatest success.

Body Image/Eating Disorders

One day, several years ago, I had an enlightening experience. I was going to see a photographer to inspect the result of a shoot. Because it happened to feature *me,* I was anxious about the results. I was going to see shots of my body, in which I wore nothing but briefs. They were the first that I'd ever seen of myself in which I was "scantily clad."

When I reached the photographer's studio, his assistant asked me to wait. "Joel will be out in a minute," she said. "He shouldn't be very long. He wanted for you to see these, though, before he wraps up his shoot."

She pointed to several large photographs that had been tacked to a board on a wall. I could see that they were of someone's physique, and whoever it was looked great. I noticed that they had been artfully cropped, to emphasize parts of his body, and were mostly of various muscle groups that were taken from different angles.

"What do you think?" Joel asked me, as soon as he entered the room.

"These pictures are great," I said shyly, "but where are the pictures of me? To be honest, I'm kind of embarrassed and scared to see how they all turned out. I'm concerned that, compared to this guy, I won't look nearly as good."

"You're kidding, right?" Joel said, in response. "These photographs *are* of you. I was hoping that you would like them—I wasn't sure what you would think. If you want, we can do a reshoot, if they're not what you had in mind."

I would never have guessed in a million years that those photographs were of me. But here's the part that surprised me most, the part that I'll never forget: When I realized whom I was looking at, my perspective completely changed. The longer I stared at the photos, the worse I believed I looked. My mind started warping the images right from the moment I knew they were me. Suddenly, all that stood out to me were my numerous "obvious" flaws. It was in that very moment that I gained a whole new point of view. For the first time ever, I truly perceived how a thin person "sees" that they're fat. From that moment on, my thoughts about image disorders have not been the same.

As I started to see these disorders pop up with increasingly more of my clients, I started to look more closely at ways to address body image concerns. Despite the fact that I learned quite a lot, and applied what I learned in my practice, most of the people I ventured to help were at first throwing me for a loop. For example, one girl almost had me convinced that she actually was in good health, despite the fact that at five feet four, she weighed only ninety pounds. Her act was so brilliantly managed and planned that I just couldn't argue her points. Not only did she have her story down, and an answer for all of my questions, she proved to be better at lying than most people are at telling the truth! It took some time, and some patience, for me to discover that I'd been duped. Seldom are anorexics ever coaxed or talked out of their problem. The problem is usually one that has a strong biochemical root.

This doesn't mean that I think anorexics should be treated only with drugs. But it does mean, in my opinion, that it's often the treatment of choice. Here's my rationale for this, based on what I've observed:

Eating disorders can threaten one's life if for too long they go unresolved. It's risky to spend a whole lot of time talking out such a serious problem, especially if someone is sinking fast, or during treatment is slow to respond.

Those who have eating disorders tend to be skilled at performing their "act." They can even fool many therapists into believing they're on the right track.

Research suggests that eating disorders have a genetic link, that the problem is *physiologic* as much as or more than it is in the mind.

Typical Signs and Symptoms of Anorexia Nervosa

- The fear of appearing fat even when at, or below, normal weight
- A persistent, staunch refusal to maintain an appropriate weight
- A distorted view of one's shape or size, perceiving oneself as fat
- For women, the absence of three or more consecutive menstrual cycles (amenorrhea)
- Weight loss of 15 percent or more of one's normal, healthy weight

Typical Signs and Symptoms of Bulimia Nervosa

- Recurrent binge eating episodes for three months, at least twice a week
- A feeling of losing control that occurs both before and during a binge
- A persistent concern with one's body, physical image, and overall size
- Regular use of laxatives or diuretics to lose weight
- A compulsion to work out excessively to offset or prevent gains in weight
- Self-induced post-binge vomiting (on a regular basis) to purge

Typical Signs and Symptoms of Body Dismorphic Disorder (BDD)

- Despite more than adequate muscle mass, a perception that one is too small
- A focus on singular body parts that are thought to be lacking or flawed
- An obsession with physical training, to the point that it threatens one's health (leads to the use of steroids or obsessive-compulsive acts)
- Comparing oneself continually to those who are "better" developed—watching those who train at the gym to size up the com-

petition, or studying photos in magazines to obsess about how one compares

When I first gave some thought to this subject, I wasn't sure how to proceed. Initially, I thought I'd add a quiz, like I have for some UFOs, but I worried that if I did so, it would not get a valid response. For example, if some of the questions were, "Are you frail?" or "Are you too thin?" a person with anorexia might answer no when she should answer yes. Whether it's how we perceive ourselves, or the facts with regard to our health, the way we tend to distort things often prevents a truthful response.

There are questions, though, that can be asked, that necessitate honest replies. For example: Have you ever binged and made yourself physically sick? Have you ever purged immediately after consuming a heavy meal? Are more than a few of your friends concerned that you look too frail or thin? Have you ever tried using laxatives or diuretics to lose weight? If you're female, have you ever missed three consecutive menstrual cycles? Is your current weight 15 percent less than the average for your frame and height? If yes is your answer to even just one of these very important questions, then your issues around food and image, without question, are UFOs.

Overcoming an Eating or Image-Related UFO

FACE THE FACTS

If you're starving yourself, or failing to eat in a way that's nutritionally sound, it's possible that you'll lose some weight—but you won't lose very much fat. Also, if you lose too much weight you'll end up *more out of shape*. Because you'll lose lots of muscle your fat burning rate will decrease and you'll find it a lot more difficult to burn calories and lose fat. In addition, starvation diets can harm your body in serious ways. An electrolyte imbalance or, for women, a lack of menstruation (amenorrhea), may result in some physical problems that can be serious if they're ignored (heart rhythm problems, a hormone imbalance, weakness, or chronic fatigue).

In addition, if you'd like to lose weight, and to do so you starve and/ or purge, in a sense it's like using a Band-Aid to cover a large, gaping, life-threatening wound. Your method of solving the problem will "help" for only a very short time. If you don't stop the bleeding and care for the wound in a sound, systematic way, it's certain to get infected and over time cause you even more pain. The steps you take in the short term to achieve an idealized goal may eventually lead to UFOs, like depression, mood swings, and fatigue.

MEDICAL INTERVENTION

Sometimes this is tricky. People with eating disorders aren't often open to treatment with drugs. Most are concerned that by taking them, they're likely to start gaining weight. Moreover, quite often subconsciously, they don't really want to be cured. They'd rather keep being obsessed with their weight, for fear that if "cured," they'd get fat. Although these are misconceptions, hearing this rarely helps. Regardless of what they are told, in their mind they remain convinced of the "facts."

People with eating disorders are also inclined to be very sly. For example, if they're prescribed a drug, and it's one that they're wary of taking, they often claim to be taking it when in fact they actually aren't. They *say* they are, to avoid any conflict with those who're concerned for their health.

If this sounds like you, it's important that you enlist some professional help. But you must seek a skilled psychiatrist who is familiar with these disorders. Remember, once you've been treated and you're back on the road to good health, you'll not only feel a lot better but you'll *look* a lot better too.

COUNSELING

The key to making this work for you lies in finding the right kind of match, connecting with someone you're able to trust who is open to how you feel. An experienced mental health counselor can give you the kind of direction you need. If medical treatment is warranted, she'll assist you in making that choice. If it turns out that counseling *is* what you need, she'll help you make that choice too. Most of all, she'll empathize with the way you think and feel. Rather than shame or pressure you, she'll offer you strength and support.

SUPPORT GROUPS

Eating disorder support groups are a great way to gain perspective. Because those who attend these groups have concerns that are very much like your own, you'll be able to trust that you won't be judged or made to feel out of place. By hearing what others have to say, you'll feel less confused and alone. Support groups help lay the groundwork for your long-term emotional health. (See Appendix for resources.)

LEARNING AND REINFORCING UNCONDITIONAL SELF-ACCEPTANCE

This is the most important, and often most difficult, thing you must do. The key to resolving disorders that involve both image and food is learning to fully accept yourself, in spite of your limitations. Again, a great way to accomplish this is by using TFT (see Chapter 1). Affirmations (like those in Chapter 1) can help as well, as can gaining perspective, either through counseling or via groups.

Lack of Time, Motivation, and Discipline

When I think about all the excuses I've heard from those who don't work out, the one that goes at the top of the list is, "I can't seem to find the time." Here's where I could be hard-hearted and tell you that this is a wimpy excuse. Or I could give you biased advice about how you should plan your time. Or I could say, "If Oprah has time, then surely, you have the time too." But I know you've heard things like this before, and it won't help to hear them again. So the only thing that I will say might be a hard thing for you to hear: If you don't have the time to exercise, it's because you're not *making* the time.

Why aren't you making the time? Most likely, the reason is this: Something you either don't know or won't say is acting as some sort of block. It could be a fear of failure, such as a fear of not reaching your goals, or it could be an old, conditioned belief, like your job must always come first. Or perhaps you have little desire to work out, even though you insist that you do. Maybe your obligations aren't what's really been holding you back. Subconsciously, you may not want to commit to the process of getting in shape. Not having time may be your excuse to avoid what you don't want to do. It's likely to be a *symptom*, not the *source*, of your actual problem.

I've found, in addition, that people are prone to define themselves by their "faults." For example, many folks seem to believe they're inherently uninspired. They also claim to lack discipline or the patience to persevere. If you, too, feel that you lack these things, consider this point of view: There are *reasons* you've lacked the follow-through, patience, discipline, focus, and drive. Being busy, or lazy, or lacking willpower aren't tendencies etched in your genes. Unlike your bone structure, foot size, or height, these are things that you can change. The fact that you've struggled in various ways doesn't mean you have "bad DNA." But it could mean that you're arranging your time to avoid doing things that are hard.

Still, some people are adamant that they're helpless to alter their fate. From "I have five kids" to "I work all day," the excuses I've heard are all old. It doesn't help much to suggest to folks that they exercise with their kids, or that training for just ten minutes a day will help them to do better work. It makes me wonder what people would do if the stakes were suddenly raised. What if the deal was you *had* to work out or your health would fail or *you'd die*? Then would you reconsider your stand about whether you had enough time? The point here is that you'll never find time if you don't give more thought to your health. If you don't move it close to the top of your list, you'll *waste* time on less crucial things.

So what is the solution, then, if it's true you're not making the time? The key to finding the time to work out is exposing your UFOs. Often when people aren't making the time, it's really because they're reversed. While consciously they may want to find time, subconsciously they really don't. Perhaps you, too, aren't finding the time for reasons you don't even know! If you've been depressed, for example, and you've buried yourself in your work, perhaps you're being limited more by your *mood* than you are by your job. If this is the case, once you realize this and acknowledge your "real" UFO, you'll stop citing work as the problem and be more inspired to address *how you feel*. When you do, you'll start to gain energy and become more inspired to work out. And you'll find, while this all is happening, that you're suddenly making the time.

One of these days is none *of these days.*
—ENGLISH PROVERB

Top Twenty-Five Excuses People Give for Not Working Out

25. The equipment I need is too costly.
24. I already get enough exercise (taking care of the kids, mowing the grass, doing housework, etc.).
23. I'm not very disciplined.
22. I'm afraid I'll run into my ex or someone I don't want to see at the gym.
21. I don't have anything to wear.
20. My body doesn't respond to exercise.
19. I'd rather do something fun.
18. I'm afraid I'll quit.
17. I can't afford to join a gym.
16. I'm too tired, I don't have the energy.
15. I'm too busy working, playing, socializing.
14. Working out is boring.
13. I'll be embarrassed and/or intimidated.
12. I'm afraid I'll injure myself.
11. I'm afraid I'll get too muscular and intimidate all of my friends.
10. There's no room in my home for the equipment I need to work out.
9. My (mother, best friend, partner, dog) prefers me the way I am.
8. I'm too old to start exercising.
7. People will think I'm vain.

6. My kids will make fun of me.

5. My (coworkers, siblings, partner, friends) will be jealous if I get in shape.

4. I need to lose some weight first.

3. I'm not in good enough shape yet to think about getting in shape.

2. I'm not a very good athlete; I'm awkward, clumsy, and weak.

1. I haven't got any time.

Biochemical UFOs

Common Health Disorders That Can Limit Your Fitness Potential

I like to exercise, but it's not always possible with my hectic sleep schedule.

—Unknown

This chapter helps you identify biochemical UFOs. I call them this because, by and large, with regard to these types of problems, a physiologic imbalance is the main, underlying cause. These UFOs, which include PMS, sleep disorders, and SAD, while fueled by emotional issues, have hormonal or chemical roots. For example, even though PMS affects how one thinks and feels, its cause relates to one's hormones more than it does to dysfunctional thoughts.

Don't fear the word "biochemical"; it's rarely as bad as it sounds. From time to time, we're all biochemically "off" to a certain degree. But when an imbalance is chronic, or is a problem you can't control, it's important for you to address it so that it won't be a UFO.

As you read through the stories that follow, consider how you may relate. Perhaps they will change how you look at yourself and the way that you view getting fit.

Attention Deficit Disorder (ADD) as a UFO

Rob, who hadn't worked out for some time, was anxious to get into shape. So anxious, in fact, that once he made up his mind to enlist my help, he called me at home, at least two or three times, on the morning of New Year's Day! When I *finally* answered his message (as soon as I checked my machine), he wanted to know why it took me "so damn long" to return his call.

"I'm serious," Rob determinedly said. "I'm ready to do what it takes. I want to get started as soon as I can, to strike while the iron is hot!"

When I questioned Rob to learn more about how I might be able to help, I was struck by the fact that although he was bright, he seemed to be very confused. After speaking to him for an hour or so, I had no clear sense of his goals. He continued to talk in circles, as if totally lost in his thoughts. He was also extremely restless, as if he'd had too much caffeine. In fact, if I hadn't inquired about this, my guess would have been that he had.

When we met at the gym to exercise, his demeanor was much the same. When I tried to give him direction, he had a habit of looking away, as if it was almost a struggle for him to look at me straight in the eyes. And although he actually did proceed to ask some relevant questions, he usually interrupted me well before I could give a reply. Moreover, Rob ignored me when I attempted to give him advice. Whenever I tried to position him in a better or safer way, he behaved like I was constricting him, as if he'd been put on a leash. He was fidgety, lax, and impatient, and beginning to get on my nerves. No matter how much I encouraged him, Rob wouldn't do the right thing. As a result, I wasn't surprised that he failed to accomplish his goals.

As I thought about what might be up with Rob, I considered the following theories: (a) Rob couldn't hear very well; (b) Rob was busting my chops; (c) Rob really liked coffee; or (d) Rob had ADD. As it turned out, he was diagnosed to be suffering from ADD. Alas, a sane explanation for the enigma I knew as Rob.

I referred Rob to a physician who was familiar with ADD. After it was confirmed that he had all of the classic symptoms, Rob was prescribed a stimulant drug that would improve his concentration. After this, when we met at the gym, he behaved like a whole different person.

He was considerably more attentive and noticeably more relaxed. Where before whenever I offered advice he instantly tuned me out, now he seemed to be nodding a lot as if what I told him made sense. Amazingly, he was agreeing with almost everything that I said.

Before Rob responded to treatment, we had worked together for months. During that time, he ignored my advice and kept falling short of his goals. But once he was treated for ADD, he started to make progress fast. In only one month, he lost eight pounds and greatly increased his strength. Six months later, he reached all his goals and was thrilled by what he accomplished—not just with regard to his health but also at work and at home. In addition, he started to do more things to take better care of himself. For Rob, being treated for ADD was his ticket to optimum health.

◆ **EXERCISE** ◆

Is an Attention Deficit Affecting Your Fitness Focus?

Put an X next to each statement that directly applies to you.

—— I often forget to perform or finish some parts of my routine (I often forget to warm up and stretch before I go out for a run).

—— More often than not, I procrastinate about dieting or working out.

—— When I work out, I am accident-prone, in particular at the gym (I often drop or trip over things, like dumbbells, machines, or weights).

—— I resist attending to details that are critical to my success. I don't want to have to think too much about anything I do.

—— My attention span tends to be limited; I have trouble taking direction (for example, taking my trainer's advice or following through with instructions).

—— Usually, when I *do* follow through, I'm inclined to hyperfocus (by using my "tunnel vision," I'm able to block things out).

—— I often begin a program feeling hopeful and inspired but find that within a very short time, I no longer feel the same way.

—— I tend to be very disorganized; I find that it's "painfully" hard to plan and follow a structured routine.

—— I'm reluctant to engage in tasks that require sustained attention; I tend to avoid activities that require concentrated effort (for example, working out in the gym or trying to change how I eat).

—— I tend to lose or misplace things that I need in order to train.

—— I tend to get very distracted by things whenever I try to work out.

—— I tend to be absentminded with regard to my daily plans (at times, I can be so scattered that I forget about working out).

Scoring

1–2: *Your attention deficit symptoms may be related to other blocks.*

3–5: *It's possible you're being limited by some form of ADD.*

6+: *There's a better than average chance that your ADD is a UFO.* If ADD is the UFO with which you can most relate, little you do is likely to help until you're successfully treated.

◆ ◆ ◆

Typical ADD Symptoms

- Impulsivity
- Restlessness
- Lack of inhibition (at inappropriate times)
- Poor follow-through
- Short attention span
- Problems with organization
- Irritability
- Impatience
- Poor judgment
- Often too trusting, sometimes naive (enticed by gimmicks and fads)
- Muddled, unfocused thinking
- Insensitivity
- Problems with short-term memory
- Fidgeting
- Often easily bored
- Long-winded manner of speaking
- Hyperactivity (sometimes)

Top Ten Ways to Identify and Overcome ADD

1. *Find a medical doctor who has ADD expertise.* If you have an attention deficit, and your symptoms have been severe, your doctor may give you the option of taking (when needed) a stimulant drug. Ritalin and Cylert are the drugs that are generally prescribed, but antidepressants, like Wellbutrin, can also be of great help. If the prospect of this is unsettling to you, there are many alternative treatments (herbs, vitamins, energy work, cognitive/behavioral therapy), but stimulants, when used judiciously, will often work faster and better. In addition, they are now widely used for *adults* who have ADD. In fact, when used correctly, their benefits can be profound. Paradoxically, those who do well on these drugs (who clearly have ADD) find that they feel *more focused, centered, positive, and relaxed.* These drugs aren't likely to work this way if you don't have ADD. So if you decide to take them, and they make you feel anxious or "revved," you're probably either on the wrong drug or attempting to treat the wrong thing.

2. *Consider enlisting the services of a holistic health professional.* Before you draw any conclusions about yourself (and/or ADD), be sure to get some opinions from those with varying points of view. For example, speak first to a therapist or a clinical dietitian (just be sure that whoever you see is familiar with ADD). There may be a way that you can be helped that you otherwise might overlook.

3. *Find out if your ADD symptoms are rooted in some other UFO.* Other types of UFOs that have symptoms of ADD include: unipolar depression (forgetfulness, low self-esteem, fatigue, poor concentration); bipolar depression (manic-depressive disorder); hyperthyroidism (anxiety, restlessness); chronic fatigue syndrome (varied symptoms); premenstrual syndrome (mood swings, inconsistent motivation, poor focus, low energy); food and environmental allergies (restlessness, irritability, fatigue, muddled thinking); anxiety disorders/stress (restlessness, irritability, tendency to fidget); and energy imbalances (varied symptoms).

4. *Sit in on a support group.* Refer to the Appendix to locate a group near you. Hearing what others have to say will give you much-needed perspective.

5. *Educate yourself.* Ask a health professional to recommend some ADD books. Subscribe to an ADD newsletter, or do research on the Web. Locate an ADD "chat room" or create a group of your own. The info you need is out there if you're ready and willing to look (see Appendix for resources).

6. *Find an "ADD coach."* Locate a person who's had ADD who is willing to be your "coach." Make sure, though, that whoever it is has been treated and had some success. It's best to hire a *professional* coach who's familiar with ADD. Professional coaches are more in tune with the issues you're likely to face and can refer you, if it's appropriate, to those who can give you more help. Refer to the Appendix to locate an ADD coach near you.

7. *Accept that your problem is apt to have roots in a neurologic condition.* Don't fool yourself into thinking that you should have the will to change. If your ADD is primarily caused by the way your body is wired, you can't just *decide* that you're going to try harder to change (or to hide) how you are. If it *is* a medical problem (which more often than not is the case), the use of a drug, like Ritalin, is probably your best bet. If you've always believed that these kinds of drugs are dangerous (or just for kids), be sure to talk to your doctor so he or she can address your concerns. It's common to have misconceptions about what these drugs can and cannot do.

8. *Determine your ADD profile.* Do you tend to accomplish more when focused on only one thing at a time (for example, training at home, alone, in a quiet, undisturbed place)? Or do you get more done when your mind is focused on more than one task (for example, riding the exercise bike, at the gym, while watching TV)? Usually, people with ADD find that one or the other is true.

9. *Remember, it's normal to feel "let down" after reaching a fitness goal.* Many who suffer with ADD are inspired by the thrill of

the quest. When a goal is achieved, they miss the excitement of facing a difficult challenge. Pursuing a goal is what fuels them; achieving a goal leaves them flat. This often results in a subconscious need to go back and begin at square one. What happens is that just before, or as, they accomplish a goal, they begin to exhibit behavior that undermines everything they have achieved (overeating, skipping workouts). If you can keep this fact in mind, and put it all into perspective, you'll begin to arrest this pattern and feel more rewarded by your success. Once you've been treated for ADD, and your reflexes start to change, you should find that before very long these "downs" begin feeling more like "ups."

10. *Contact an organization for additional information.* Refer to the Appendix to locate a group near you.

Seasonal Affective Disorder as it Relates to Getting Fit

Seasonal affective disorder, also known as SAD, is a much underrated problem with regard to getting in shape. In fact, more than half of my clients suffer from symptoms of SAD. Fifty percent! Of course, living in New England, SAD tends to be more common. Thankfully, though, most people weather the gloom without long-term effects. Although they do tend to gain some weight and spend less time working out, they're rarely affected to such a degree that they find themselves wholly off track. Most of them suffer from something that's better described as the winter blues. But for others, it's very clear that SAD is a major concern. When winter arrives and the sun starts to hide, they feel as if they should hide, too. Actually, for the most part, they behave a lot like bears. They fill up on food, retreat to their caves, and sleep pretty much until spring. They also tend to get mighty upset when I venture to wake them up.

For 15 percent of my clients, SAD is a UFO. Every year, as the winter draws near, they experience similar symptoms. Like clockwork, they start sleeping more, moving less, and finding themselves gaining weight. They also tend to feel more depressed and to crave lots of carb-laden foods. In addition, their sex drive decreases and they tend to withdraw from their friends. Add to the list reduced energy, and SAD's UFO link is clear. If you have SAD and ignore it, or fail to see how it's a block, you'll find that at the same time every year you'll struggle to stay in good shape.

Strangely, SAD doesn't only occur in the winter or fall. Some people only have symptoms of SAD in the summer or spring. But this is usually only the case for a small percentage of people. Most people who suffer from SAD feel worse when they're getting less light.

Now my clients with SAD know exactly what they must do. Before they start having symptoms, which is usually late in the fall, they begin using artificial light to replace what they lose during the day. Most sit about three feet from a box that provides them with full-spectrum light (the typical strength of this light is 2,500 to 10,000 lux). They find that sitting in front of this box for at least twenty minutes each day awakens the part of their brain that shuts down in the winter when there is less sun.

A light box isn't the only way to get full-spectrum light. Some prefer using light visors, so that they don't have to sit in one place. In fact, I know people who wear them when they are running or working out. Regardless of what the light source is, the difference it makes is astounding. Most of my clients *look forward* to winter now that they're using bright lights. They don't gain weight, they don't crave carbs, and they rarely avoid working out. Some of them actually make better gains in the winter than during other months! If you too suffer from SAD, it's time to wake yourself up. Perhaps what you learn as you read this book will help you to "see the light."

◆ EXERCISE ◆

Is Your Motivation to Exercise Being Affected by SAD?

Put an X next to each statement that directly applies to you.

―― My motivation to exercise always wanes in the winter or fall.

―― I always crave carbohydrates more during the fall and winter months.

—— Without fail, every year, I gain more than five extra pounds in the winter or fall.

—— I'm *much less* inspired to exercise on cloudy or overcast days.

—— I typically have more energy during the spring and summer months.

—— I sleep a lot more in the winter and fall than I do during the summer or spring.

—— I'm inspired to work out more consistently if I'm routinely exposed to the sun.

—— I'd usually rather remain indoors during the fall and/or winter months.

Scoring

  2: *You may have the winter blues.*

  3+: *It's likely you have SAD.* Be sure to consider what follows regarding ways to address this problem.

◆ ◆ ◆

Three Ways to Identify and Overcome SAD

1. *Consult with a doctor or therapist who has SAD expertise.* Refer to the Appendix to contact an SAD expert near you.

2. *Full-spectrum bright light therapy.* To determine the treatment protocol that will benefit you the most, consult with a health professional who's well versed about SAD. He or she will suggest to you the best ways to use bright lights. The angle at which the light hits your eyes (as well as its lux or brightness) is tailored to meet your personal needs and adjusted if they should change. The length of time you're exposed to the light is a critical factor as well. While some people need an hour or more, for others, ten minutes is fine. Moreover, studies have verified that we do absorb light through our skin. By exposing the light to an area where you tend to have thinner skin (behind the knee), the result can be the same as viewing light (from a box) with your eyes. Consult an SAD specialist to determine which options are best. (See the Appendix for sources from which you can purchase full-spectrum lights.)

3. *Schedule some winter vacations in a place with a warm, sunny climate*. In places that have more winter sun, SAD is less common.

Ways That Premenstrual Syndrome Can Be a UFO

"Ricky!" Lucy abruptly shrieked, as if she were being attacked. "Have you seen my brand-new running shoes, the ones with the bright blue trim? I can't seem to find them anywhere! So much for my afternoon jog . . ."

"Lucy, honey," Ricky replied, "you shooz iz right on you feet! Heh, heh, heh, heh, heh, heh, heh. Just wait 'til Fred hears 'bout this!"

"Don't tell Fred, you insensitive creep. Then Ethel will know," Lucy barked. "To her, it'll be just one more thing that proves that I've lost my mind. In fact, when I saw her yesterday on my way to work out at the gym, she actually had the nerve to suggest that people who jog are insane! She's probably right—I guess I'm crazy to think it'll do any good. I mean, every month it's the same old thing, the same old depressing result. As soon as my hormones get out of control, like clockwork I start gaining weight! And some help you are, you drum-pounding dork, you don't ever help me at all! I've begged you to let me perform at the club, but you won't even give me a chance. Please Ricky, *please* let me dance with your band. I know it would help me lose weight!"

I'm always amazed that so few of my clients make links to their PMS. In spite of the fact that their symptoms have been consistently throwing them off, most never guess that PMS has kept them from reaching their goals. Over and over again, I hear them repeat the same old tale: "I seem to do well for a couple of weeks, and then I get way off track." When I ask if when this happens they feel more cranky or more fatigued, they often say something like, "Yeah, so what? All women have PMS. I don't see it slowing down others that much, so why should I let it stop me?" "Do you have PMS right now?" I ask. "Is that why you seem so miffed?" (which at times has prompted an angry tirade from a soon-to-be-former client). Some women can't see how *their* PMS could prevent them from reaching their goals. They dismiss the idea PMS that their PMS might, in fact, be affecting them more.

The point here is that PMS may hinder you more than you think. As most women tend to experience it, it's not a significant problem, at least not in terms of the impact it has on their efforts to get into shape. In fact, on a scale from 1 to 10, if 10 is extreme PMS, most of my female clients would probably score between 1 and 6. For others, though, this syndrome occurs to a markedly greater extent. Women who score between 7 and 10 have what is called PMDD (premenstrual dysphoric disorder). For them, it's far more important that something be done to address how they feel.

◆ EXERCISE ◆

Is Premenstrual Syndrome Keeping You from Achieving Your Fitness Goals?

Put an X next to each statement that describes the way you feel.

—— My energy level consistently drops, quite a bit, when I have PMS.

—— In a steady, predictable pattern, my mood swings affect what I do. I notice that when I have PMS, I have less desire to work out.

—— My cravings are often profoundly worse when I suffer from PMS.

—— I don't like attending to details when I experience PMS. The routine things I have to do are always more of a hassle, especially when they involve concerns that in some way are workout-related.

—— I often begin eating poorly at the same exact time every month; I'm rarely able to eat well during the time that I have PMS.

—— Often, when I'm premenstrual, I avoid interacting with others (I find myself avoiding the gym or skipping my walks with friends). I'm often so thin-skinned and edgy that I take what they say the wrong way.

Scoring

2+: *Look into your PMS.* See your physician soon for advice about how to relieve your symptoms. You might be surprised to discover the difference the right type of treatment can make.

◆ ◆ ◆

Signs and Symptoms of PMS That Act as UFOs

- Abdominal bloating and cramping
- Anxiety
- Back pain
- Breast pain and swelling
- Confusion
- Problems with coordination
- Depression
- Severe and frequent mood swings
- Fatigue
- Bingeing
- Headache
- Insomnia
- Irritability
- Joint pain and swelling
- Lethargy
- Nausea
- Sugar and salt cravings
- Sinus problems
- Light-headedness
- Emotional instability
- Withdrawal from family and friends

Common Nutritional Factors That Contribute to PMS

- *Excessive consumption of foods that contain refined sugar and/or flour*
- *Frequent consumption of dairy products*
- *Too much caffeine* (from sources including soda, coffee, and chocolate)
- *Vitamin B_6, B_{12}, C, E, magnesium, and selenium deficiencies* (required for the adequate breakdown of estrogen in the liver)
- *A diet high in animal fat* (increases prostaglandin F2 and overall estrogen levels; decreases progesterone levels)

Common Emotional Factors That Contribute to PMS

- ◆ *Unresolved emotional issues, body-centered traumas, holding onto emotions rooted in difficult past events*
- ◆ *Stress that results from relationships that are abusive, unstable, or strained*
- ◆ *A recent traumatic experience* (for example, a death in the family)
- ◆ *Dysfunctional family history* (for example, alcoholism)

Common Physiological Factors That Contribute to PMS

- ◆ *A high body fat percentage.* An excess of estrogen (estrone) can be linked to a surplus of fat.
- ◆ *Seasonal Affective Disorder (SAD).* A predisposition for SAD can exacerbate PMS symptoms (your PMS symptoms are apt to be more severe in the winter months).
- ◆ *Going off birth control pills*
- ◆ *Childbirth or the termination of a pregnancy*
- ◆ *Low blood levels of progesterone* (a hormone that offsets estrogen)
- ◆ *Inactivity*

Top Ten Ways to Stop PMS from Being a UFO

1. *Eliminate caffeine.* For those whose PMS is severe, caffeine makes symptoms worse. Even one cup of coffee can have dramatic, adverse effects and often exacerbates symptoms that are already causing you stress.

2. *Consider vitamin supplements.* According to Christiane Northrup, M.D., effective PMS supplements include these important components: magnesium (400 to 800 mg.); B complex (50 mg.); borage oil, black currant seed oil, or evening primrose oil (as directed on the bottle). In addition, she suggests a diet high in complex carbohydrates (primarily vegetables and whole grains, or nutritious foods low in fat).

3. *Increase calcium intake but emphasize nondairy sources.*

4. *Give yourself a daily dose of bright, full-spectrum light.* This means exposure to natural light or a source you can use in your home (see Appendix). Viewing the light first thing when you wake can often quell PMS symptoms.

5. *Investigate natural progesterone.* Ask your physician if this could help to control your PMS symptoms. Because it isn't routinely prescribed, it's not always easy to find, so if it's not at your pharmacy, ask where else you should look. Contrary to what is typical with synthetic forms of this drug, natural progesterone's side effects are usually less severe. In addition, premenstrual headaches often respond particularly well.

6. *Perform cardiovascular exercise at least three times a week.* The challenge is trying to do it when you're depressed, upset, or fatigued. Here are a few suggestions if you find that this is the case:

   ◆ *At first, just keep it simple, don't plan to do too much.* The easier exercise is at this time, the more likely you are to do it. Walking is often the ideal choice for those who have PMS. It's simple to do, easy to start, and doesn't involve undue stress. Other forms of exercise may be uncomfortable during this time, especially if they involve heavy lifting or rapid, high-impact movements. This is a time to go within, to nurture and comfort your body. It's *not* the time to subject yourself to very high levels of stress.

   ◆ *Try not to plan a specific length of time that you "have to" work out.* Be a lot more flexible with regard to whatever you do. For example, if you're taking a walk, rather than plan twenty minutes, tell yourself that you're just going to go as far and as long as you can. Do as much as you comfortably can, and it won't seem so much like a chore. Always respect how your body feels, in particular during this time.

7. *Try using these acupressure points, both before and during your cycle. Rushing Door:* in the center of the crease where your upper thigh meets your lower torso; *Sea of Energy:* on your

lower abdomen, two finger widths under your navel; *Gate Origin*: on your lower abdomen, four finger widths under your navel. While applying moderate pressure, and while using your fingers or thumb, hold each point for a minute or more and repeat until symptoms subside.

8. *Consult a holistic nutritionist for advice about herbs that may help*. Herbs that can be helpful for relieving PMS include dong quai/damiana, chaste tree berries, cramp bark, echinacea, and bilberry. Teas that are often suggested include chamomile, burdock root, licorice, red raspberry, dandelion, and fresh ginger root.

9. *Find out if antidepressants are an option that you should consider*. Selective serotonin reuptake inhibitors (SSRIs) such as Prozac, Zoloft, and Paxil have proved to be helpful for two out of every three women who have PMS. "Severe PMS is a disorder," says Ellen Freeman, Ph.D., codirector of the PMS program at the University of Pennsylvania. "To argue that it shouldn't be treated is like saying that we shouldn't treat depression."

10. *Ask your doctor about using drugs that suppress ovarian function*. Researchers at the National Institute of Mental Health have found that leuprolide, a drug that retards the production of progesterone and estrogen, can help reduce PMS symptoms.

Sleep Disorders as UFOs: More Common Than You Think

Sam approached me years ago, as he said, "at the end of his rope." He claimed to have trouble breathing, in particular when he worked out. In addition, whenever he exercised, he quickly became fatigued. So besides having problems with breathing, Sam was perpetually pooped.

Even his medical doctors didn't know what to make of his plight. "I can't figure out what's wrong with me," Sam complained, in a frustrated tone. "I've had lots of tests and read lots of books, but nothing I've tried has worked. Have you ever heard of a problem like this or known someone else like me? Why is it that when I exercise, it's so hard for me to breathe?"

I then asked Sam some questions that, apparently, no one else had. "Does your wife complain that you snore," I asked, "and if so, is it often and loud? Do you suffer from allergies, sinus pain, headaches, infections, or frequent colds? Are your breathing patterns abnormal at night, off and on, when you're trying to sleep? Does it sound like you're sometimes holding your breath, or gasping, as if you need air? Do you wake up feeling unrested, groggy, or dazed, as if in a fog?"

"Yes to all of those questions," Sam replied, with a puzzled look. "As a matter of fact, it's rare that I ever feel like I've had enough sleep. At any rate, the doctors I've seen aren't convinced that it's any big deal. Still, no matter what anyone says, I *know* I've got some kind of problem."

I first referred Sam to a specialist for some tests on his nose and his throat. I then sent him to a doctor who was an expert on problems with sleep. After he met with both of them, he was scheduled for routine tests. The tests were performed at a sleep lab at a hospital close to his home. During the night he spent at the lab, he was monitored while he slept, and technicians recorded the data required to determine the cause of his problem. Sam had obstructive sleep apnea, which confirmed what both doctors suspected. As it turned out, it was causing his problem with breathing and poor, restless sleep.

Sleep apnea is a condition resulting in labored, unsteady breaths. People who have this disorder usually don't even know that they do. When they're "asleep," their breathing actually stops for brief spurts of time, depriving their body of oxygen and preventing good-quality sleep. Often, it's caused by a nasal bone "split" (deviated septum) that contributes to some type of block. Usually it's congenital, but it can result from a break. Either way, it's a problem that causes more trouble than most people know.

To confirm his diagnosis, Sam was hooked to a CPAP device (continuous positive air pressure), which is basically just an oxygen mask that connects via tubes to a tank. By means of the CPAP, pressurized air was forced past his nasal obstruction. Because Sam's breathing was much improved while using the CPAP device, it served as further proof that he'd been correctly diagnosed.

When Sam started using the CPAP at home, his whole life began to change. He slept through the night with no trouble at all and woke up feeling clear and refreshed. And to his surprise he observed that for once he could finally breathe, not only much better in general but, in particular, when working out. Suddenly he could exert himself without always gasping for breath. Not only was he less winded, but he also was less fatigued.

As Sam made continued progress, he decided to go one more step. He elected to have nasal surgery to address the real source of his problem. After he had the procedure he couldn't believe how much better he felt. He also found that he no longer needed the CPAP in order to sleep. By correcting his nasal obstruction, he accomplished the same result. Moreover, his weight very quickly dropped and his stamina greatly increased. In fact, he said that he couldn't remember a time that he ever felt better.

Working with Sam gave me insight into a broad range of problems with sleep. It made me begin to look into this more when I started to work with new clients. I was shocked by the number of clients I had who were not getting adequate sleep. I also learned that insomnia was only one of many sleep problems. Over the course of fifteen years, while working with hundreds of people, at least 10 percent of my clients revealed that their sleep cycles were out of sync. These people, whom some call "larks" or "owls," were "up" when they should have been "out." Their sleep cycles weren't in harmony with the way they were forced to live. Larks have what's called (in technical terms) an "advanced sleep phase syndrome," which basically means that their "time clock" has been set for an early rise. Conversely, owls have "delayed sleep phase," which means that they go to sleep late (after 1 A.M.). Both have circadian rhythms that reach their peak at inopportune times. Their body's internal time clock doesn't jive with societal norms.

How can something like this be related to problems with getting in shape? It's simple. In fact it's so simple that many are blind to the fact that it's true: People are too often pushing themselves to work out at unfavorable times! Their energy level and mental state, as well as their concentration, are not even close to what they must be to enable continued success. This is akin to someone who functions quite well on a "normal" schedule rising at 3 A.M. every day to make himself go to the gym. Your mind and body cannot perform at your mental and physical peak if your physiological time clock says, "Right now, you should be asleep." Variables like your temperature or your preworkout BMR (basal metabolic rate) may not be set at a high enough point to enable an optimum start (your body temp is much lower at times when your body "should be" asleep). It's much like trying to start your car on a very cold winter day. If your engine isn't warmed up enough, you're likely to sputter or stall. In this way, this type of problem is without question a UFO.

◆ EXERCISE ◆

Are Your Fitness, Strength, and Energy Being Restricted by Restless Sleep?

Put an X next to each statement that directly applies to you.

—— I rarely wake up feeling rested. My energy level is low. I yawn and feel groggy most of the day. Exercise feels like a chore.

—— I prefer to stay up late at night, even when forced to rise early.

—— When the only time I can exercise is *before* I go to work, whenever I try to do so I'm usually too fatigued.

—— Although I'm an early riser, in the morning I can't work out (I fear that I might disturb someone, or the gym at that time is closed).

—— I have been told that I snore a lot, mainly when lying faceup.

—— My breathing is loud and/or labored sometimes, and when training the problem is worse.

—— I find it hard to focus because I seldom get restful sleep (when I work out, it's hard to concentrate—my fatigue affects how I think).

Scoring

1–2: *If your problems are significant and observed on a regular basis, it's important that you see a specialist to determine the primary cause.* When it comes to sleep, even one or two things can turn out to be UFOs.

3+: *There's a better than average chance that your problems with sleep are UFOs.* The sooner that you address them, the sooner they'll stop being blocks. See a sleep doctor as soon as you can to get to the root of your problem.

◆ ◆ ◆

Insomnia

Classic symptoms:

- ◆ It takes you more than thirty minutes most nights to fall asleep.
- ◆ You awaken five or more times most nights before you plan to rise.
- ◆ The amount of time you're awake during the night is more than thirty minutes.
- ◆ The time that you're asleep most nights is six and a half hours or less.
- ◆ The duration of your slow-wave sleep is fifteen minutes or less. (Slow-wave sleep is the third and fourth stage, or theta and delta wave, sleep. It's known for its curative properties and for its role in maintaining good health.)
- ◆ Your symptoms cause you to feel fatigued or groggy most every day.
- ◆ One or more of these symptoms has persisted for three or more weeks.

TOP FOUR WAYS THAT INSOMNIA CAN BE A UFO

1. *Causes reductions in energy and, when training, rapid fatigue.* Studies reveal that sleep debt can affect your athletic performance. One study showed that when losing sleep equivalent to one night, it takes *less time* (11 percent) for your muscles to tire when you train. Another study, involving a group of male and female cyclists, revealed that a loss of sleep forced them to work harder when they worked out. After having three fewer hours of sleep on the day before they worked out, the subjects had higher heart rates than they normally did when they trained. In addition, all of the subjects had a reduction in oxygen uptake and increased

concentrations of lactate that were measured in samples of blood. This made them fatigue at a much faster rate and caused them to have less endurance.

2. *Reduces motivation and causes procrastination.* You feel much less like working out if you're always extremely fatigued. Telling yourself that you're tired becomes a very convenient excuse.

3. *Poor or insufficient sleep can affect your rate of recovery.* When you don't get enough good-quality sleep, your body is under more stress. As a result, you don't get the rest you need for your body to thrive. Your muscles don't have enough time to "revive" before you must train them again.

4. *It is much harder to concentrate on workout-related details.* A consistent lack of quality sleep prevents you from being focused. You tend to pay less attention to things that are critical to your success (for example, using proper technique or maintaining a proper position).

Top Ten Ways to Prevent Sleep Debt from Being a UFO

1. *Practice good "sleep hygiene" every night before you retire.* Never climb into bed until you're good and ready to sleep. Do what you can to block out or remove any noise that will keep you awake. Develop a personal ritual that consistently helps you relax (for example, listening to music, meditating, or reading a book). Make sure that your bedroom (especially your bed) is arranged for your optimum comfort.

2. *Try using acupressure to release your sleep-hindering blocks.* The following points, used one at a time or in any combination, can often be very effective as a means to achieve better sleep. *Third Eye Point:* directly between your eyebrows, where your forehead meets your nose; *Wind Mansion:* in the hollow at the base of your skull, low on the back of your head; *Spirit Gate:* directly on the wrist crease, in line with your little finger; *Joyful Sleep:* on the inside of your lower leg, below where your

ankle protrudes; *Calm Sleep*: on the outside of your lower leg, below where your ankle protrudes. Push firmly with comfortable pressure, close your eyes, and try to relax. Hold each point for a minute or more and repeat—if you're still not asleep.

3. *Go to bed consistently at the same time every night.* Don't get into bed, though, if you don't feel like you could sleep. In other words, don't force yourself if you're still feeling wired or stressed. Wait until you feel tired enough to let go and fully unwind.

4. *Never eat or drink too much before you go to bed.* Allow four hours between heavy meals and the time you get into bed. Although your insulin level spikes right after you've had a large meal, it also *decreases* dramatically within a very short span of time. This often causes anxiety, twisting and turning, and/or restless legs. Avoid sugar, salt, caffeine, nicotine, and foods that are high in fat. In addition, drinking too much may result in repeated trips to the john. Try not to eat or drink anything that could wake you or stress you at night.

5. *Try using TFT.* Refer to Chapter 1 for information on TFT (thought-field therapy). If the "things on your mind" are keeping you up, and you can't escape negative thoughts, TFT can alleviate them and help you to get better sleep.

6. *If you're taking a drug, have your doctor adjust the timing, dose, and/or type.* Inform your doctor if physical symptoms (headaches, anxiety, or persistently restless legs) keep you from getting good sleep. You may need to change the dose you're on to relieve or prevent side effects. Or, a different drug could be a less problematic choice. Whatever the case, don't ever assume that your symptoms are all in your mind. If your doctor "adjusts" the drug you're on, or prescribes one that works a lot better, any symptoms you currently have are likely to disappear.

7. *Avoid any mental or physical stress before you hit the sack.* Put off or shun all discussions that have the potential to cause you stress. For a change, try turning the news off and instead going straight to bed. It may be that more than you realize, your subconscious absorbs what you hear.

8. *Consult with your doctor to see if there is a primary, unexposed cause.* A physiologic disorder can be at the root of deficient sleep. Your insomnia may be a symptom of a veiled, underlying condition (for example, a nasal obstruction).

9. *Try using sleep aid supplements (e.g., melatonin) and/or modifying your diet.* Avoid the use of sleeping pills, unless for a very short time. They decrease REM (rapid eye movement) sleep and interrupt normal sleep patterns. Ask your doctor if melatonin could be a viable option and if there're any concerns you should have (if you're on other drugs). Although it's still controversial, melatonin has shown promise. But it should not be considered an option that doesn't present some risk. It should not be taken haphazardly or without your physician's okay. In fact, some doctors have found that lower doses (1 mg. or less) work best. In addition, a good dietitian will make you aware of what foods to avoid. He or she will advise you about how to eat to allow for good sleep.

10. *Try using herbal or vitamin supplements prior to going to bed.* Herbs that can sometimes be helpful include chamomile, Siberian ginseng, licorice root, valerian, scullcap, St. John's Wort, lemon balm, and passionflower. Vitamin supplements also can help, including calcium, magnesium, pantothenic acid, inositol, GABA (to stabilize glucose levels), and B_1 or Niacinimide (for nightmares). An alfalfa tonic is worth a try, as well as a light bedtime snack (for example, a small banana). Don't try anything, though, without first getting your doctor's approval. If they're not taken correctly, supplements could do more harm than good.

Sleep Apnea

Classic symptoms:

- Loud, persistent snoring that tends to be worse when you're on your back.
- Snoring that's louder (in general) after consuming alcohol
- Night sweats

- Cessation of breathing when sleeping for very brief lengths of time (typically, one to ten seconds)
- Hypertension
- Erratic, labored breathing and choking or gasping for breath
- Nasal congestion that's worse in bed or frequently under exertion
- Frequent headaches and daytime fatigue; typically groggy when waking
- Restless behavior when sleeping (tossing and turning in bed)
- Frequent nighttime arousals
- Sufferers often are out of shape or noticeably overweight

THREE COMMON WAYS THAT SLEEP APNEA CAN BE A UFO

1. Your blood absorbs less oxygen, which can lead to daytime fatigue.
2. It can cause labored breathing when training.
3. It's often a cause of sleep debt, which if ongoing or severe can make you fatigue at a much faster rate whenever you try to work out. In addition, it lengthens recovery time between each successive session.

TOP TEN WAYS TO MINIMIZE OR OVERCOME SLEEP APNEA

1. *Raise the head of your bed.* By elevating your mattress at the top, where you rest your head, you may find that it's not quite as difficult to breathe comfortably when you sleep.
2. *Use a flat pillow or neck roll when you're lying in bed on your back.* If your neck or head is bent forward, it's usually harder to breathe.
3. *Lose some weight.* If you really do have sleep apnea, and you also are overweight, it might be a struggle for you to lose weight until you've addressed your problem. But if you can, despite the fact that it's likely to be a challenge, you may find that as you start losing weight, you also start *gaining* sleep.
4. *Stay away from alcohol or drugs with sedative effects.* Studies suggest that alcohol actually makes sleep apnea *worse*. Sedatives (such as Valium) and, at times, antihistamines, have also been found to increase the number of apnea-related events.

5. *Identify and avoid food and/or environmental allergens*. Allergy testing can help you to know if you're feasting on sleep-hindering foods (for example, foods with tyramine, such as aged cheese, chocolate, sauerkraut, wine, bacon, ham, sausage, eggplant, potato, spinach, and tomato). Tyramine will prompt the release of a chemical called norepinephrine, which by stimulating your body actually keeps you from falling asleep.

   You should also find out if allergens are affecting you while you sleep. In fact, your bed and your bedroom are apt to attract and to harbor dust, which may lead to breathing problems that could prevent you from getting good sleep. An air filter or air ionizer is an option that's likely to help.

6. *Sleep on your side (and not on your back)*. Sew or tape a tennis ball to whatever you wear to bed, attaching the ball so it contacts your skin near the center of your upper back. That way, if you turn onto your back, the ball will make you turn over.

7. *Don't smoke*. Smoking, for obvious reasons, can make breathing problems worse.

8. *Try nasal decongestants*. Consult with your doctor for guidelines about what type will work for you best.

9. *Try ginkgo biloba*. This extract of a Chinese tree may increase blood flow to the brain. In addition, it's believed to aid in oxygenating the blood. As such, it could quell the fogginess caused by apnea-related events.

10. *If your symptoms are clearly chronic, or have been diagnosed as severe, continuous positive air pressure (CPAP) or nasal surgery may help*.

Nocturnal Myoclonus (Restless Leg Syndrome)

Classic symptoms:

- ◆ Restless, crampy, or twitchy legs before and/or while you're asleep
- ◆ A compulsion to move or to shake the legs, as if they're about to cramp
- ◆ Difficulty falling asleep

TWO COMMON WAYS THAT RESTLESS LEGS CAN ACT AS A UFO

1. It prevents good-quality sleep and limits your energy when you're awake.
2. It's apt to keep you from falling asleep, increasing your level of stress.

THREE WAYS TO TAME RESTLESS LEGS

1. *If you're taking a medication, try a new type or new dose.* It's possible that the drug you're on is exacerbating your problem. Some studies show, for example, that Prozac makes restless legs worse. If your legs have become more restless since being put on a new kind of drug, consult your physician to get some advice about how to adjust what you take.
2. *Ask your physician if taking a drug is warranted in your case.* Klonopin is often prescribed to stifle restless legs. Other drugs can be used as well, so be sure to consult your physician.
3. *Vitamin E at bedtime and folic acid may help.* According to many homeopaths, this helps to prevent restless legs. Some suggest taking 400 IU of vitamin E before bed, as well as 800 mcg. of folic acid per day. Again, before you start doing this, it is wise to consult your physician.

Advanced Sleep Phase Syndrome

Classic symptoms:

◆ A predisposition to fall asleep very early (before 8 P.M.)
◆ Waking up well before you plan to rise and begin your day
◆ Feeling extremely groggy or tired when up after 8 P.M.

Delayed Sleep Phase Syndrome

Classic symptoms:

- ◆ A tendency to wake and rise unusually late in the day (after 10 A.M.)
- ◆ A tendency to fall asleep unusually late in the evening (after 2 A.M.)
- ◆ Feeling groggy or very fatigued long after an early rise

TWO COMMON WAYS THAT SLEEP PHASE PROBLEMS CAN BE UFOS

1. *When working out, your body and mind can seldom perform at their peak.* Your physiological time clock conflicts with societal norms.

2. *Times that work best for working out have a tendency not to work out.* Training is less convenient at the times that you're most awake.

THREE WAYS TO ADDRESS AND OVERCOME AN ABNORMAL SLEEP/WAKE CYCLE

1. *Chronotherapy.* By shifting your wake time or bedtime each day, either forward or back *by one hour,* your circadian rhythm (or "time clock") can be reset for a different cycle. If you normally wake at noon, for example, but have to get up at six, each day you set your alarm clock *back* to wake at an earlier time.

2. *Full-spectrum, bright-light therapy.* Bright light has been used with great success to modify patterns of sleep. There are various ways to accomplish this, so you should seek professional help. Typically, you are exposed to bright light at the time you desire to rise. If you tend to rise at 10, for example, and you'd rather get up at 8, you turn on the light at 8 A.M. upon waking from your alarm. Conversely, if you'd like to stay up but have trouble staying awake, you would use the lights in the evening before you plan on going to bed. Bear in mind that when using the lights,

regardless of time of day, the strength of the light is a factor, as is the angle at which it is viewed (most light sources are rated at 2,500 to 10,000 lux). Consult with a sleep/wake specialist to determine what works best for you. (Refer to the Appendix to find a list of bright light sources.)

3. *New evidence shows that your cycle can change when exposing bright light to your skin.* One study shows that by shining bright light on a spot behind either knee, some people notice results that compare to viewing bright light with their eyes. The advantage is that your eyes can be closed while you're resting or lying in bed. In addition, the light can be helping you while your eyes remain fixed on your work.

Common Hormonal Imbalances That Could Be Acting as UFOs

A hormone imbalance can hinder your health in ways you're not likely to know. Deficiencies often cause problems that lead to bone loss and loss of strength, as well as fatigue, reduced energy, and diminished resistance to stress. Most people regard these kinds of things as typical for their age. But as we age and see that our bodies do not work the way they once did, perhaps instead of accepting this we should try to identify why. Perhaps there is something that we can all do to offset our "predestined" decline.

Before you start thinking that hormone replacement will cure you of all of your ills, in the words of an infamous president, let me make this perfectly clear: if you have a hormonal imbalance, and it's truly a UFO, replacing what's lacking with more than you need may do you more harm than good. Studies do clearly show, though, that hormone replacement can help, *if* you have a deficiency *and* you take the right drug and right dose. But depending on who you ask about this, it may or may not be an option. Not all physicians are fully convinced that the pros outweigh the cons. With this in mind, if you think there's a chance that you could be hormone deficient, be sure to get several opinions before you choose a medicinal course.

DHEA (DEHYDROEPIANDROSTERONE)

DHEA is a hormone that we all produce less as we age. Although technically it's a steroid, it's not like the kind that builds strength. It comes mostly from our adrenal glands, as well as our brain and our skin. For most, this hormone is at its peak around twenty years of age. By the time we get to be forty, though, we produce only *half as much*. This may be part of the problem for some who are struggling to get into shape.

Low levels of DHEA are linked to a number of physical changes. Besides a reduction in energy that for some can be quite severe, low levels of DHEA can often make body fat harder to lose. Some even think that when levels are low, we age at a much faster rate. According to William Regelson in his book *The Superhormone Promise*, every adult who's at least forty-five can be helped by DHEA. But although it's widely available and can be purchased without a prescription, it will only be of some value to you if your levels are currently low. A blood test or a saliva test is the best way to know where you stand.

TESTOSTERONE

Testosterone is a hormone abundantly present in young adult males. But for roughly one-third of all middle-aged men, testosterone levels decline—enough to affect their health in a way that prevents them from getting fit. Common deficiency symptoms include (in addition to lack of libido) decreases in strength and muscle mass, marked energy loss, and fatigue. Depression, frail bones, and premature aging are typical symptoms as well. Postmenopausal women also experience a decline, which often results in depression or a diminished desire for sex.

Hormone-replacement therapy often can be a viable option, but *only* if you take testosterone to restore *normal*, healthy levels. Studies show that this hormone, when prescribed and used the right way, can combat depression, prevent heart disease, and improve your overall strength. In particular, you should consider this if you're fifty or more years of age, but bear in mind that at any age you could have deficiency symptoms. For those who find themselves "breaking down" at a faster than normal rate, a testosterone deficiency could very well be a UFO.

Moreover, of special importance for women concerned about fragile bones, testosterone can prevent bone loss for those who are postmenopausal. Anything you do to increase the density of your bones can help you to be less injury prone as well as a great deal stronger.

Testosterone, when used in amounts that exceed what a person needs, can cause a whole rash of symptoms that range from depression to loss of hair. Fortunately, the dose that's required is generally very small, not nearly enough to cause any serious, long-term adverse effects. To determine if taking testosterone is an option that you should consider, a routine saliva or blood test can be arranged through your medical doctor.

HUMAN GROWTH HORMONE (hGh)

This hormone is still controversial with regard to medicinal use. A number of studies have shown, though, that for some, when used the right way, it has age-reversing properties that can greatly improve one's health.

The pituitary gland makes most of the hGh that our body needs. Although it increases dramatically during the growth spurts of our teens, it declines at a rate of 14 percent every decade of our adult life. Deficiencies of hGh can cause a loss of bone, as well as a breakdown in muscle mass and significant loss of strength. It can also cause depression and increases in body fat. As a result, it's possible that for some it's a UFO. If you've noticed that you're more frail and fatigued than the norm for someone your age, you might want to have your physician test your levels of hGh.

While older adults may want to consider how hGh might help, bear in mind that the jury is really still out regarding this drug. There has not yet been enough research performed to support its commonplace use. In addition, a higher than normal dose can cause a whole rash of symptoms (see Chapter 3). But if you have any cause to believe that you're hGh deficient, it certainly wouldn't hurt to consult an expert on hormone replacement. He or she will evaluate you to determine if it is an option. At the rate that research is being conducted on hormones like hGh, perhaps by the time you read this new findings will color your choice.

THYROID

For some people, hypothyroidism can be a UFO. An underactive thyroid gland is the cause of this disorder, the symptoms of which can range from fatigue to a slow metabolic rate. Conversely, the term *hyperthyroid* means that one's thyroid is working too hard. The symptoms are muscular weakness, profuse perspiration, and palpitations, in addition to weight loss, bulging eyes, and reduced tolerance to heat. This problem is much less common, though, and less often a UFO.

Thyroid hormone "ignites" the fuel that's created and used by our cells. This fuel, which is called ATP (or adenosine triphosphate) is created by mitochondria, which are like tiny cellular engines. These engines, as they burn oxygen (and as a result, create ATP), provide the fuel or the energy that supports all our bodily functions. To perceive how thyroid hormone aids in the energy/fuel-making process, imagine it's much like the starter fuel that is used to light coals on a grill. In a sense, this hormone lights up the coals that allow our "cell engines" to run.

When we don't have enough thyroid hormone to properly fuel our cellular engines, free radicals are created by all of the oxygen that isn't burned. Damage caused by free radicals is linked to a number of serious problems, such as cancer, heart disease, cataracts, arthritis, Parkinson's, and diabetes. In this way, a thyroid deficiency can be a serious threat to one's health.

Thyroid deficiency symptoms also can keep you from getting fit. When your thyroid is underfunctioning, you burn less fat than you should—a fact that is frequently cited by those who consistently battle the bulge. If you've been inclined to use this excuse, it's important to keep this in mind: If your metabolic rate is slow, and you've found it hard to lose weight, hypothyroidism isn't the only possible cause. Often, when people are slow to burn fat, the thyroid is falsely accused.

If you truly are thyroid deficient, you could have a number of symptoms. For example, you may be fatigued, depressed, or unable to move at full speed. You may also have hearing loss, hair loss, chills, cold skin, and frequent infections. Add to the list slow speech, poor memory, and swelling around the face, and it's easy to see how this problem could be a serious UFO.

It's also worth noting that diet pills can often be thyroid unfriendly. They deplete the thyroid of iodine, which it needs to perform its job. Ironically, if you take diet pills in order to burn more fat, your thyroid gland will start slowing down and you'll actually burn *less* fat. Because thyroid hormone functions, in part, to keep metabolic rates stable, when the thyroid gland lacks iodine, metabolic rates decline. Pollutants and various allergens can also play a part, as can X rays and a lack of vitamins A and E (or zinc).

For those who are over fifty years old, thyroid dysfunction is common. It occurs in one out of twenty men and one out of every ten women. But even if you're a bit younger than this, a thyroid test wouldn't hurt. In fact, Johns Hopkins researchers say that for those over thirty-five, thyroid testing should be made a routine part of yearly exams.

Clients of mine whose symptoms caused me to suspect they were thyroid deficient often complained that what bothered them most was failing to lose any weight. But this fact alone, in and of itself, didn't signal a thyroid problem. They also had many other common thyroid deficiency symptoms. If this sounds like you, there may be a chance that you really are thyroid deficient, but to gain a more accurate sense of this, you might want to try this test: Put a thermometer under your arm as soon as you wake, while in bed. If your temperature is normal, you're apt to have good thyroid health. If after at least ten minutes it's still below 97.4, it's possible that your thyroid gland is failing to do what it should.

If you think that you're thyroid deficient, you should consider a thyroid test. If the test confirms that you need it, you can take thyroid medication, or perhaps desiccated thyroid, often considered a more "natural" choice. This will allow you to burn more fat and to be at your best when you train. In addition, there are some supplements that can contribute to good thyroid health (CoQ10, Vitamin A, B complex, E, zinc, taurine, raw iodine, kelp), but you may want to talk to a homeopath to determine which options are best.

... 6

Physical UFOs

Exposing Fitness Obstacles with Physiological Roots

If you don't get everything you want, think of the
things you don't get that you don't want.

—Unknown

This chapter examines UFOs with physiological roots. By revealing physical UFOs that you may not know you have, it
guides you to conquer the personal blocks that have kept you from
reaching your goals. It begins by revealing the blocks that result from
musculoskeletal problems and explains how these blocks can be overcome by improving your spinal health. By learning how "subluxations"
limit your strength and your range of motion, you'll see how improving
your posture can be a key to achieving your goals. You'll also learn how
your environment can affect how you feel when you train and ways that
pollutants and chemicals may be restricting your physical strength. In
addition, you'll see how allergens such as mold, pollen, ragweed, and
dust could, more than you even realize, limit your energy when you
work out.

Also in this chapter, by looking at common prescription drugs,
you'll see how typical side effects could be acting as UFOs. Lastly, by
looking at body types, like Pitta, Vata, and Kapha, you'll learn how
these classifications are used to predict your best exercise options. As
you gain a sense of how physical limits can often be predisposed,

you'll learn to reframe how you see them and begin to draw more from your strengths.

How Musculoskeletal Problems Can Be Common UFOs

Shawn was a weight-lifting novice with competitive aspirations. At five feet nine, 210 pounds, he was solid and powerfully built. But as hard as he worked at improving his lifts, he could not make additional gains. He feared he'd reached his potential and that his strength would never improve.

When I questioned Shawn about how he worked out, it seemed that he did the right things. He tried different cycles and different techniques, but little he did seemed to help. But as I learned more, I began to suspect that Shawn had a different problem. I could see, as I noticed his posture, that his spine was excessively arched. It also appeared, when he stood up straight, that his pelvis was tilted, or sloped. When I measured the span from the top of his hip to the floor (on both sides of his body), I found that the length of his right leg was an inch longer than his left. I wondered if this was affecting him in a way that restricted his strength.

I suggested to Shawn that his posture might be what was impeding his gains. In addition, I strongly suggested that a good chiropractor would help. He agreed that it seemed like a good idea and contacted one that he knew. At first, he was scheduled for X rays and routine diagnostic tests. Then, when he met with his doctor to get an update on his results, he was told he had scoliosis and some misaligned bones and joints. At this time, he went into treatment, which continued for several months.

As the condition of Shawn's spinal health improved, and his joints became better aligned, he noticed a vast improvement in his energy level and strength. With the aid of a lift that he wore in one shoe to even the length of his legs, he no longer had all the stress on his spine that he did when his hips were askew. Moreover, the curve in his spine, with regular treatment, became less pronounced, and the adjustments I helped him to make with his form and posture were of great help. Only three months after Shawn received his first chiropractic treatment, his bench press increased by thirty pounds, and his other lifts jumped as well. By aligning his spine and his joints in a way that reduced all the stress on his nerves, his muscles responded immediately by greatly increasing in strength.

As soon as I witnessed what happened with Shawn, I went to see Dr. Jon Berg, an experienced chiropractor with a background in fitness and health. I figured that if he could resurrect Shawn, perhaps he could help me, too.

When I went to see Dr. Berg he took several X rays of my spine. When he showed them to me, I could see very clearly the ways it was misaligned. Because I'm aware of the value of freeing up energy blocks in the body, the theory behind chiropractic made an enormous amount of sense. By adjusting misaligned vertebrae or appropriate parts of the body, nerves and energy channels can be relieved of stress-induced blocks. These blocks can be caused by emotions or by trauma to parts of one's body. A vertebral misalignment, often called a subluxation, can limit your strength and energy, not to mention your overall health. For many of those I've worked with, they've clearly been UFOs.

Although I had fewer problems than Shawn, there were still some I had to address. Once I did, before very long, my strength levels greatly improved. I also became more limber and felt more energized when I worked out. As soon as I had this experience, I was prompted to share it with clients. Now I routinely do postural screens and tests to evaluate strength. I also check ranges of motion when I suspect a particular problem. I certainly can't diagnose anyone, but I do know when something is wrong. And now, when there is, I no longer fret about where to refer my clients.

Is chiropractic an option that could possibly benefit you? If you jog, run, walk, do aerobics, use steppers, or frequently play active sports, the odds that you have subluxations (or misaligned joints) are extremely good. The stress that you place on your back and your knees, in particular, may cause you trouble. For example, one of my clients discovered that when she put stress on her knees, she couldn't work out as long or as hard as she could when she did other things. But a few simple knee adjustments proved to be of tremendous help. Once her knees were correctly aligned, she no longer had any pain.

If you often work with computers, bicycle, "spin," or lift heavy weights, a chiropractic adjustment can ease the stress on your hands and your wrists. Often repetitive stress injuries, such as carpal tunnel syndrome, are a problem for those whose work involves repetitious physical tasks. This includes clerical workers, cashiers, programmers, hairstylists, and painters, as well as assembly line workers, mechanics, plumbers, musicians, and dentists. In addition, these types of activities tend to put stress on your neck and your back. If, whenever you exercise, you have pain in these stress-prone areas, you may need to adjust your spine as much as you do the way you train. The point here is that stiffness, pain, or a limited range of motion can be caused by a subluxation, which is not difficult to treat. Just like with anything else, though, you need to consult the right person. If you're able to open your mind a bit, I think you'll be glad that you did.

◆ **EXERCISE** ◆

Have Subluxations or Misaligned Joints Been Acting as UFOs?

Put an X next to each statement that directly applies to you.

—— My bones and joints are unstable, especially when I work out.

—— I have pain in my back, my joints, or my neck fairly often when I'm working out.

—— I've been told that I have scoliosis, but I haven't addressed my problem.

—— I've been told that I have lordosis (swayback), but I haven't addressed my problem.

—— I have pain that radiates down my leg that is worse when I'm working out.

—— When I perform certain movements, they always cause me pain.

—— When performing certain movements, I have a limited range of motion.

—— My posture tends to be very poor, especially when I work out.

—— Impact-related stresses bother my knees, ankles, feet, and/or back. I can't keep them up very long without feeling tired or being in pain.

—— I often perform activities that put stress on my hands or wrists (for example, typing, riding a bike, rowing, or lifting weights).

—— In the past, I suffered an accident that caused trauma to parts of my body (for example, an auto accident or an injury playing a sport).

—— I run, jog, or walk with an uneven gait, bowlegged, knock-kneed, or hunched up.

—— When I train with weights, my movements are usually quick, uncontrolled, and explosive. I try to lift as much weight as I can, without much regard for my posture.

—— I shrug my shoulders and arch my back a lot when I'm working out.

Scoring

1–3: *If your problems are common or serious, it's important that they be addressed.* Seeing a good chiropractor is an option that you should consider.

4+: *The odds are good that you have UFOs that relate to your subluxations.* With the help of muscle tests, X rays, and routine diagnostic procedures, you should have all of the data you need to decide on a curative course.

◆ ◆ ◆

Chemical, Seasonal, and Environmental Allergies

When Peter first came to see me, he appeared in excellent health. And, compared to most folks, he appeared to have few UFOs. He was focused, inspired, and disciplined, and determined to reach his goals. Still, he accomplished few of them, despite doing everything right. He worked very hard and gave it his all but still achieved modest results.

Peter had me baffled. The only thing that gave me a clue that something peculiar was wrong was that often he felt light-headed and even lethargic when he worked out. He had asked his doctor about it but was told that he checked out fine. It was obvious, though, that something was wrong, and it clearly was slowing his gains.

One day, Peter revealed to me that he'd been laid off from his job. Because of this, we agreed to limit our sessions to once a week. Several weeks later, he noticed his body improving in leaps and bounds. At first, I wondered if Peter was following somebody else's advice. To my relief, when I asked about this, he assured me it wasn't the case. Then, I deduced that the stress of his job had been greater than he'd let on.

He assured me, again, that this wasn't true and that losing his job stressed him more. Then it finally occurred to me to ask what his job involved. Peter worked in a chemical plant, in a warehouse, surrounded by toxins. More than he ever imagined, they were hazardous to his health. Besides causing various symptoms that were vague or hard to describe, the chemicals drained his energy and made him feel poorly when he worked out. Once he stopped being exposed to them, his UFOs disappeared.

Now I know how important it is to ask about someone's surroundings, whether it's in relation to where they live *or* where they're employed. I never fail to address this now whenever I work with new clients. Some are beauticians or hairstylists who work with hair products and sprays, many of whom are clueless about why they feel sluggish whenever they train. Others are cosmetologists who work with or sell perfumes. A few are manicurists, for whom nail polish causes a problem, and some paint houses or work every day in body shops, spray-painting cars. But most of my clients can best be described as "electromagnetically ill." Many spend hours each day in front of computers, staring at screens. Electric field radiation, and the glare produced by these screens, causes headaches, drowsiness, vision disturbances, energy blocks, and fatigue. Seldom do people realize the way this affects them when they work out. By the time they get to the gym, *if* they do, their energy level is low. Their exposure to radiation, in effect, is a UFO.

Oftentimes, even the gyms themselves are environmentally "flawed." For those allergic to dust, for example, gyms are a hazardous place. Typically, dust builds up around high-traffic areas, mats, and machines. For those who are allergic to dust, this can affect how you train, as you may tend to cough and wheeze a lot or find it a struggle to breathe. If you want to increase your energy and be more focused when you work out, you may need to change your environment or learn new ways to address your concerns.

Common chemical allergens include exhaust fumes, asbestos, and gas, as well as radon, or formaldehyde (if you work in a research lab). A chemical allergy starts when toxins are stored within fatty tissues. The more you're exposed to chemicals or to environmental pollutants, the more your body responds to the threat by trying to build a defense. When your body detects contaminants, histamines are produced, resulting in allergy symptoms such as skin rash and ringing ears. Other symptoms include feeling dizzy, energy loss, and fatigue, as well as a slowed metabolic rate, infections, headaches, and the runs. These are all things that could limit you when you're trying to get into shape. If you have three or more of these symptoms and live or work in a hazard-prone place, it's important to see an allergist to determine the root of your problem.

Seasonal allergies often result from mold, pollen, ragweed, and dust. These types of allergies tend be worse when your body contains excess mucus, which often occurs when your body becomes allergic to certain foods. The mucus you have in your body actually harbors seasonal irritants, so if you have seasonal allergies, you should test for food allergies too. As your body reacts to an allergen, your free radical levels increase, which reduces your antihistamines and can lead to liver dysfunction. In addition, adrenal exhaustion can trigger a number of allergy symptoms, as can being allergic to yeast, and a lack of "healthy" fat (essential fatty acids).

Seasonal allergy symptoms include sore throat and sinus infection, as well as headache, coughing attacks, and a stuffed up or runny nose. Additional symptoms include skin rash, asthma, or even insomnia, as well as hypoglycemia and occasionally menstrual disorders.

Thirty-five million Americans are chronic allergy sufferers. I've found, through my work as a trainer, that it's the case for one out of five. Although many people have allergies that are transient, mild, or infrequent, chronic allergy sufferers tend to have serious, long-term problems. It's this group of people who typically find that their allergies are UFOs.

◆ EXERCISE ◆

Are Chemical/Seasonal Allergies Frequently Acting as UFOs?

Put an X next to each statement that directly applies to you.

—— I often have trouble breathing when I work out in a dust-prone place.
—— I work around dangerous chemicals and potentially toxic fumes.
—— I notice that allergy symptoms often occur when I'm working out.

—— I struggle exerting myself outdoors (for example, I wheeze when I jog), especially when there's a weather change, or during certain times of the year.

—— My home's heating unit is fairly old and has not been checked for leaks.

—— My allergy symptoms are often worse when inhaling or breathing smoke.

—— My basement is cluttered and dusty, as are certain parts of my home.

—— My home contains insulation that is very old or exposed.

—— Excessive amounts of asbestos are in places throughout my home.

—— I spend lots of time in a place with lead paint, and often it contacts my skin.

—— My heating and air-conditioning vents have never or rarely been cleaned.

—— My car is an older model, and the heat-A/C system is poor.

—— I spend lots of time in traffic, frequently stopped behind buses or trucks.

—— I live or work in a city that has significant problems with smog.

—— I live in a part of the country where the weather is inconsistent.

—— I live in a part of the country where the humidity tends to be high.

—— I often use perfume, cologne, hair spray, or scented health products and soaps.

—— I wash my clothes with products containing chemicals I don't need.

Scoring

1–3: *You're exposed to various allergens that could possibly be UFOs.* See your physician or allergist to find out if you need to be treated.

4–7: *You may have specific allergies or a condition that's making them worse (asthma, PMS).* You may work, live, work out, or spend lots of time in a place that is causing you problems.

8+: *It's likely that you have multiple chemical/seasonal sensitivities.* Until you address your allergies, you may never be optimally fit. Your symptoms will limit you to an extent that prevents you from reaching your goals.

◆ ◆ ◆

Top Ten Ways to Conquer Chemical/Seasonal UFOs

1. *Investigate new research findings and ask about new types of treatments.* In the past, allergy sufferers had to have many shots every year. Researchers now have discovered new ways to limit how many you need. Allergy Immuno Technologies, a California-based research company, has developed a course of treatment that involves having far fewer shots. In addition, at the National Institute of Allergy and Infectious Diseases (NIAID), scientists have performed studies linking some allergies to our genes. The ultimate cure for allergies, according to NIAID researchers, may lie in specific gene therapies that are tailored to meet our needs.

2. *Avoid eating mucus-enhancing foods, like sugar, caffeine, and milk.* Avoid dairy products in general, in addition to processed food. For at least seven days, abstain from *all* of these foods to eliminate toxins. Emphasize non-mucus-forming foods, like vegetables, fruits, and whole grains. Changing the way you eat may be the best thing you can do, whether to halt your allergies or to help them to be less severe.

3. *Take appropriate supplements to build up your body's defenses.* Supplements that can be helpful include B complex and CoQ10, as well as omega-3 flax oils and ascorbate vitamin C. An adrenal or raw thymus supplement may be of help to you as well, so consult a holistic practitioner for advice about what works best. Remember, there's not one prescription that works in the same exact way for us all. The type and dose of whatever you take must be tailored to meet *your* needs.

4. *Consult with an expert who knows about herbs to determine if they might help.* A naturopath or homeopath, or a good holistic physician, should be able to give you guidance about different ways to make use of herbs. Gingko biloba is often prescribed for those who are allergy-prone, but garlic, echinacea, and bilberry may be helpful to you as well. While you do have a number of options, it's best not to choose them yourself. Be sure to consult a professional who can provide you with sound advice.

5. *Use Coca's Pulse or a muscle test to assess your allergic response.* (See Chapter 7 to find out more about how these types of tests work.)

6. *If you smoke, use TFT to quit.* Smoking makes allergies worse. In addition, secondhand smoke can often be just as much of a problem.

7. *Use these acupressure points, together or in combination: Middle of a Person:* between your nose and upper lip, in the hollow, close to your nose; *Heavenly Pillar:* one half inch under the base of your skull, about one inch from the center (this point can be found on the part of your neck that feels like a "ropy" muscle, on either side of the hollow on the back upper part of your neck); *Three Mile Point:* four finger widths below the knee, on the outside of the leg; *Sea of Energy:* two finger widths under your navel.

8. *Consider seeing an allergist.* He or she will evaluate you to see if you need to be treated. In addition, you may receive allergy tests to assess the extent of your problem. The results may show that your allergies limit you quite a bit more than you think. If this is the case, just taking this step could eliminate some UFOs.

9. *Change or avoid the environment that is causing your allergy problems.* For example, use a computer screen on your monitor at all times. This keeps radiation and glare from triggering UFO symptoms. In addition, have radon and water tests conducted at your home and clean out all vents and baseboards to eliminate excess dust. If your health club or gym is a dust-filled place, or the locker rooms aren't very clean, consider joining a different club, or mention it to the staff. Have your car's heating and A/C checked, to be sure they are running "clean." Make sure that when you're in your car, you recirculate the air. When in traffic, keep your outside vents closed, to avoid breathing hazardous fumes. Don't walk or run in areas where there tends to be lots of smog. Purchase an air ionizer, or an air filter, for your home. And last, whenever it's practical, keep the A/C on in your house. It will act as an allergen filter (as long as the filter is clean).

These are only a few of the steps that it may benefit you to take. By being more conscious of how your environment could be impeding your health, you'll be more inspired to make changes that will help you to be toxin-free.

10. *If you have a seasonal allergy, limit your use of drugs.* Corticosteroid drugs, when used continually over time, can depress your immune defenses and make allergens harder to fight. In addition, try not to use nasal sprays for longer than four or five days (unless your physician prescribes a type that is okay to use long term). These sprays can have a rebound effect and cease to be as effective. Often, the more you use them, the more you tend to need them. Consider using a saline spray to keep nasal passages moist. In addition, when taking allergy meds, conservative use is best. Also, if you have allergies and at the same time feel depressed, ask your physician if Sinequan is an option that you should consider. (Sinequan is an antidepressant with histamine-blocking properties.) Be sure to consult your physician if you have any other concerns.

How Common Medications Can Cause or Contribute to UFOs

For Ellen's forty-fifth birthday, she received an unusual gift, a series of sessions with me, arranged for her in advance by her spouse. When I met with Ellen, she admitted that she wasn't pleased with the way she looked. She said that compared to her girlfriends, she was "terribly" out of shape. She wondered why *they* could stick to a plan, whereas she was "such a lost cause."

"I'm not sure what's going on," Ellen said, "but I'm never inspired to work out. Not only that, but it seems like I've gained as much weight as my friends have lost! I'm discouraged because while they always seem so excited about working out, I always feel so lethargic, like it's a chore just to get off the couch. I really would like to exercise more, but when push comes to shove, I can't!"

When I asked for some background about Ellen's health, she revealed that she had hypertension. For more than a year she'd been taking a drug (propranolol) for her blood pressure, as well as a diuretic (to adjust her sodium balance). They helped keep her pressure under control and helped her to feel more relaxed.

"How do you feel overall," I asked, "now that you're taking these drugs? Have you noticed you've felt any different? Have you had any adverse effects?"

"Not really anything obvious," Ellen said, with a quizzical look. "I'm not having headaches or dizzy spells, if that's what you're worried about. I guess I should probably tell you, though, that my husband thinks I'm depressed. Sometimes I think that he might be right—compared to before, I am. But I think it's because, as hard as I try, I can't seem to lose any weight. If I just could get rid of this hideous flab, I bet I'd feel pretty good."

"I'd like you to talk to your doctor," I said, "and tell him what you just told me. I'm guessing that one of the drugs you're on is affecting the way you feel. If this is the case, it might help explain why you're struggling to get into shape."

When Ellen talked to her doctor, he was surprised to hear her complaint. He asked why it took her so long to suspect that the drugs could be causing a problem. She told him she wasn't aware that "feeling depressed" could be drug related and thought that the reason she felt so depressed was because she was so out of shape. He then started her on a different drug that would have less effect on her mood. Immediately, she felt a big change and was able to start working out. And as she lost weight, and her blood pressure dropped, she was able to lower her dose.

As Ellen's condition improved even more, she asked for a trial without drugs. Once she received her doctor's consent to wean off the diuretic, her energy level greatly improved and she felt more inspired to work out. Then, as she started to exercise more and consistently eat healthy foods, she weaned herself off of the other drug too, and still kept her blood pressure low. Adjusting her medication was the key to her newfound success.

I can't tell you how many clients I've had who were limited somehow by drugs—even common prescription drugs that are generally helpful and safe! What surprises me most of all, though, is that most never make the connection. They seem to get used to the way they feel, or they simply don't want to complain. They ignore or accept all the side effects and think they have no other choice. The point I'd like to emphasize here is that often you do have a choice. Drugs can be changed, a dose can be changed, in fact, *many* things can be changed. Don't allow needless side effects to fuel or create UFOs. If you're taking a drug, and you're not feeling right, don't be resigned to your fate. Find out from your doctor what options you have that are less apt to cause UFOs.

◆ **EXERCISE** ◆

Are Side Effects of the Drugs You Take Resulting in UFOs?

Put an X next to each statement that directly applies to you.

—— I haven't talked with my doctor about how the drug I take makes me feel.

—— I recall, looking back, that before taking drugs I didn't have so many symptoms.

—— I've noticed since I started taking a drug that my diet or workouts have suffered.

The drug that I'm currently taking seems to:

—— make me lethargic and slow.

—— increase my appetite.

—— make me feel depressed.

—— drain or restrict my energy.

—— make me feel tense or uptight.

—— make it much harder to sleep.

—— make my mouth dry when I train.

—— make me feel very fatigued.

—— make me feel dizzy when standing.

—— increase my heart rate when I train.

—— make me sweat more when I train.

—— lead to intestinal problems (bloating or gas).

—— make me feel drowsy or weak.

Scoring

1–3: *While your symptoms may or may not be caused by the drug that you are taking, it's best to consult with your doctor about any change in the way you feel.* Often, even one symptom can be enough to prevent your success.

4–6: *The type or dose of the drug you take may need to be changed or adjusted.* See your physician about this soon, to rule out or correct any problem.

7+: *The type or dose of the drug you take is clearly not serving you best.* Be sure not to make any changes, though, without first consulting your doctor. On occasion, even with side effects, a drug can help more than it hurts.

◆ ◆ ◆

Commonly Used Medications and Symptoms That Are UFOs

The following medications are those that are commonly used by my clients. They're also those that have symptoms that lead most often to UFOs. Although this list is incomplete, it's intended to give you perspective. Any drug can cause side effects that lead to UFOs.

ANTIDEPRESSANTS (SSRIs—SELECTIVE SEROTONIN REUPTAKE INHIBITORS)

Prozac (fluoxetine)
Paxil (paroxetine)
Zoloft (sertraline)
Luvox (fluvoxamine)

Possible UFO symptoms: weight gain, insomnia, agitation

TRICYCLIC ANTIDEPRESSANTS

Pamelor (nortriptyline)
Sinequan (doxepin)
Norpramin (desipramine)

Tofranil (imipramine)
Elavil (amitriptyline)
Vivactil (protriptyline)
Surmontil (trimipramine)
Anafranil (clomipramine)

Possible UFO symptoms: dry mouth, excessive thirst, weight gain, blurred vision, dizziness, heart rate irregularities

MAOI (MONOAMINE OXIDASE INHIBITORS)

Nardil (phenelzine)
Parnate (tranylcypromine)
Marplan (isocarboxazid)

Possible UFO symptoms: adverse food interactions with foods containing tyramine (aged cheese, yogurt, wine, avocado, beer, others), hypertensive crisis (dangerously high blood pressure), weight gain, dry mouth, fatigue, drowsiness, headaches, nausea, insomnia, agitation

OTHER ANTIDEPRESSANTS

Wellbutrin (bupropion)—used for depression and ADD
Effexor (venlafaxine)
Desyrel (trazodone)

Possible UFO symptoms: orthostatic hypotension (dizziness when standing), excessive sedation, weakness, nausea, dry mouth, constipation, excessive sweating

ANTIHYPERTENSIVES
Beta-Blockers
Inderal (propranolol)
Tenormin (atenolol)
Catapres (clonidine)
Aldomet (methyldopa)

Possible UFO symptoms: depression, orthostatic hypotension (dizziness when standing), fatigue, light-headedness, headaches, reduced blood flow to the extremities

Calcium Channel Blockers
Procardia (nifedipine)
Isoptin (verapamil)
Cardizem (diltiazem)

Possible UFO symptoms: depression, lethargy, apathy, orthostatic hypotension (dizziness when standing), weakness, gastrointestinal problems (diarrhea, constipation)

DIURETICS

Diamox (acetazolamide)
Diuril (chlorothiazide)
HydroDiuril, Dyazide, Diupres, Inderide, Aldactazide (hydrochlorothiazide)

Possible UFO symptoms: reduced potassium levels; weakness; dizziness; mood changes; headaches; dry mouth/thirst; irregular heart rate; fatigue; weight changes; allergic reactions (for those allergic to sulfa drugs); possible adverse reaction with tricyclic antidepressants (dangerous drop in blood pressure), as well as cortisone, alcohol, or licorice (excessive potassium loss that could cause abnormal heart rhythms)

CNS (CENTRAL NERVOUS SYSTEM) DEPRESSANTS

Antianxiety and sleep-enhancement drugs

Benzodiazepines
Klonopin (clonazepam)
Ativan (lorazepam)
Xanax (alprazolam)
Valium (diazepam)

Dalmane (flurazepam)
Halcion (triazolam)
Librium (chlordiazepoxide)
Serax (oxazepam)

Nonbenzodiazepines
Buspar (buspirone)

Possible UFO symptoms: depression, drowsiness, lethargy, fainting, tremor, blurred or double vision, gastrointestinal problems, nausea, respiratory depression

CNS (CENTRAL NERVOUS SYSTEM) STIMULANTS

Cylert (pemoline)
Ritalin (methylphenidate)
Dexedrine (dextroamphetamine)

Possible UFO symptoms: blood sugar instability, palpitations, rapid heart rate, headache, hypertension, agitation, anxiety

ANTIHISTAMINES

Claritin (loratadine)
Hismanal (astemizole)
Benadryl (diphenhydramine)

Possible UFO symptoms: agitation, tachycardia (rapid heart rate)

HYDROCORTISONE

Hydrocortisone
Cortisol

Possible UFO symptoms: diminished adrenal function, headache, gastrointestinal problems, insomnia, weakness

ANTACIDS

Tagamet (cimetidine)
Zantac (ranitidine)
Axid (nizatidine)
Pepcid (famotidine)

Possible UFO symptoms: agitation, adverse drug interactions

BIRTH CONTROL DRUGS (CONTRACEPTIVES)

LoOvral
Ortho-Novum
Triphasil

Possible UFO symptoms: depression, headache, increased or reduced appetite, nausea, bloating, muscle and joint pain, fluid retention

ESTROGEN-REPLACEMENT DRUGS

Premarin
Estradiol
Estrone
Ogen
Conjugated estrogens
Esterified estrogens

Possible UFO symptoms: depression, dizziness, irritability, appetite loss, swollen feet and ankles, nausea, diarrhea, stomach cramps

How Your Somatotype (Body Type) Can Affect How You Choose to Get Fit

Because bodies come in different shapes as well as different sizes, it seems to make sense that we should be working them out in different ways. When the way you're exercising isn't serving your body best, you're much more likely to injure yourself or to keep falling short of your goals. To illustrate, if you're very tall, full-figured, or overweight, by forcing yourself to run or jog you could cause your own UFO. Not only will you dislike it and find it a tedious, difficult task, but you're also apt to get injured due to the stress on your knees and back. Finding out what your body type is can help you to plan how you train. When you're stumped about what type of workout to do or about the best way to proceed, your body type characteristics can be a factor in making your choice.

When they're defining somatotypes, meaning specific physical types, fitness experts often refer to the following classifications: the mesomorph, a muscular build, with broad shoulders and narrow hips; the ectomorph, a more fragile build, inclined to be tall and lean; and the endomorph, a heavier build that tends to be stocky or fat. The theory is that based on a person's musculoskeletal structure, we can guess and prescribe the exercise modes that will work for that person best. Although these classifications have been widely used for years, I use the three Ayurvedic types that are favored by Eastern physicians. The body type classifications referred to as Vata, Pitta, and Kapha take into account many factors other than bone structure, size, or physique. They account for one's personal preferences, behavioral patterns, and patterns of sleep, as well as physical traits such as eye and hair color, pulse rates, and skin. In short, they're more all-inclusive and more useful for guiding my clients. According to Dr. John Douillard, in his book *Body, Mind, and Sport*, these are the characteristics that best describe Vatas, Pittas, and Kaphas.

Vata

MENTAL AND BEHAVIORAL CHARACTERISTICS

Often has good short-term memory and an active or restless mind. Quickly grasps new concepts, and focuses best on short-term goals. Tends to have active, physical dreams with light but steady sleep. Often speaks fast with a high-pitched voice and tends to eat food very quickly. Prefers warm food, has a variable mood, and tends to dislike cold weather. Is also excited quite easily and is fickle with money and friends.

PHYSICAL AND ATHLETIC PROFILE

Tends to have lighter shades of hair, which is usually medium-thick. Skin is typically dry and rough and often is darker in color. Cold hands and feet are common as well, in addition to fairly small eyes. Usually finds it hard to gain weight and tends to be lean or thin. Veins and tendons are prominent, and resting heart rates run high (usually 70–90 for men and 80–100 for women). Exercise tolerance levels are low, and strength and endurance are fair. Tends to be quick and to have good speed but doesn't like competition. Usually has a fairly small frame, is tall, and has a slight build.

Pitta

MENTAL AND BEHAVIORAL CHARACTERISTICS

Usually has a sharp intellect; is aggressive and self-inspired. Has a good memory in general and tends to have good concentration. Grasps new concepts fairly well but at a more moderate speed. Often has angry, violent dreams but does not tend to wake at night. Speech patterns tend to be short and sweet, with few extraneous words, and voices are generally medium-pitched (infrequently low or high). Tends to eat food at an average speed but is often impatiently hungry. Also prefers to eat colder foods that don't need much preparation. Moods are typically slow to change and tend to be more consistent. Does well with cooler weather and likes to have time alone.

PHYSICAL AND ATHLETIC PROFILE

Tends to have hair that is medium-thick, with reddish or light-colored hues. Skin is usually soft, moist, warm, and light pinkish-red in color. Eyes are usually average-size, with yellow- or red-tinged whites.

Weight tends to be in a normal range, and resting pulse rate is average (60–70 for men, 70–80 for women). Exercise tolerance tends to be fair, and endurance is usually good. Strength is better than average, as is foot speed and physical skill. Tends to be very competitive and attracted to active sports. Usually has a medium frame and tends to be average height.

Kapha

MENTAL AND BEHAVIORAL CHARACTERISTICS

Is usually calm and steady, with logical, organized thoughts. Tends to have good long-term memory but is forgetful in the short term. Has excellent concentration and can focus for long spans of time but takes a long time to grasp and process instructions or things that are new. Tends to have scenic, romantic dreams, and sleep is sound, long, and deep. Speech is generally slow and clear, and voice is lower-pitched. Usually eats very slowly and tends to like warm or dry food. Doesn't like weather that's damp or cool and is normally slow to excite. Tends to be frugal and practical and to have solid friendships that last.

PHYSICAL AND ATHLETIC PROFILE

Often has thicker, oily hair that tends to be dark brown or black. Also tends to have paler skin that is frequently moist and cool. Eyes are large with "glossier" whites, and teeth are typically large. Weight tends to be above average and metabolism is slow. Resting pulse rate is 50–60 per minute, in general, for men, and for women 60–70 is a typical Kapha range. Veins and tendons are often concealed, and skin is usually thick. Exercise tolerance often is high, and endurance is generally good. Strength levels tend to be high as well, but foot speed tends to be slow. Easily handles competitive stress but is not particularly driven. Can have a high percentage of fat on a large, fairly solid frame.

About one-fourth of my clients are clearly Vatas, Pittas, or Kaphas. They tend to identify strongly with one of these three sets of characteristics. For these folks, knowing their body type helps them to chart an appropriate course. It helps them to channel their energies in a much more productive way.

If you find that you have a blend of several different body type traits, your choice of options for working out is not as clearly defined. You need to rely on your instincts (or on the test at the end of this section). If you don't relate very strongly to a specific classification, I've found that it's best not to use them at all, as opposed to being unsure. While some experts cite combination of types, like Vata-Pitta or Pitta-Kapha, I've found that this tends to confuse folks more than, in practice, it really helps. But if you clearly identify with one of these three Ayurvedic types, the recommendations that follow are likely to put you on the right track.

If at least three-fourths of a certain group's traits are applicable to you, the following exercise options are most likely to suit you best.

Vata Exercise Options

Low-impact aerobics or dance
Water/aqua aerobics
Slide aerobics
Bicycling (touring)
Rowing
Hiking
Tai chi
Step machines
Elliptical cross-trainers
Swimming
Walking
Weight training
Yoga

Pitta Exercise Options

Basketball
Cycling
Skating

Kayaking/rowing
Mountain biking
Noncompetitive racquet sports
Downhill skiing
Cross-country skiing
Water skiing
Circuit training with weights and/or exercise machines

Kapha Exercise Options

Aerobics
Basketball
Bodybuilding
Calisthenics
Cross-country running
Cross-country skiing
Fencing
Gymnastics
Handball
Lacrosse
Racquetball
Rock climbing
In-line skating
Rowing
Soccer
Step machines
Swimming
Water/aqua aerobics
Tennis
Volleyball

What if you can't identify with one of the three Ayurvedic types? A fitness personality test may give you a different perspective. According to Jonathan Niednagel, author of *Your Key to Sports Success*, the key to knowing what works for you best lies in learning to "know thyself." To find the fitness activity that is best for you, he says, defining your personality type is the first, most important step. Much like the Myers-Briggs test often used for job placement and planning, the same type of test can be used to determine your best path to getting in shape. Here's an abridged variation to help you determine your best fitness options.

◆ **EXERCISE** ◆

The Fitness Typing Self-Quiz

Consider the following questions and circle the letters describing you best.

1. Introverts tend to have few close friends and enjoy spending time alone. They're often shy or uncomfortable being in social settings or groups. Extroverts like to talk a lot and feel energized when they're in groups. They tend to have many acquaintances and to feel anxious when they're alone. If you think that you're an introvert, circle the letter **I**. If you think that you're an extrovert, circle the letter **E**.   I   E

2. By nature are you intuitive (you play things by ear and you trust your "gut"), or are you sense-oriented (a literal thinker who wants to know facts)? If you think that you're more intuitive, circle the letter **I**. If you think that you're sense-oriented, circle the letter **S**.   I   S

3. Are you usually more of a thinker (mainly objective and focused on goals), or are you more of a feeler (often subjective and process directed)? If you tend to be more of a thinker, circle the letter **T**. If you tend to be more of a feeler, circle the letter **F**.   T   F

4. Do you tend to be judgmental (decisive, a planner with good follow-through), or do you think you're perceptive (more spontaneous, likes new options)? If you're usually more judgmental, circle the letter **J**. If you tend to be more perceptive, circle the letter **P**.   J   P

◆ ◆ ◆

FINDING YOUR FITNESS TYPE

Write down, in order, the letters you circled and find out your type (below).

Type I. The Structured Realist: ESFJ, ESTJ, ISFJ, ISTJ

Your threshold for pain is generally low; you rarely take risks with your body. Your body is very important to you, as is your physical image. New fitness fads attract you, and you like to try things that are new, as long as they're not too strenuous or too hard on your muscles and joints.

Favorable fitness activities: low-impact aerobics; water/aqua aerobics; swimming; jazzercise; power walking; ice skating; in-line skating; cross-country skiing; elliptical cross-trainers; short, well-structured workouts (either with free weights or machines).

Type II. The Adaptable Realist: ESTP, ESFP, ISTP, ISFP

You prefer unstructured training routines. You're impulsive and like to ad-lib. You tend to get bored very easily and need to have options when you work out.

Favorable fitness activities: skiing, in-line skating, mountain biking, jazz/funk aerobics, freestyle dance, weight training (in a gym with numerous options), rock climbing, aerobic boxing, freestyle swimming, soccer.

Type III. The Logical Visionary: EITP, EITJ, IITJ, IITP

You tend to be goal-oriented; you like a well-planned routine. You work well with personal trainers and are open to taking advice. You enjoy being active and working out hard. Your physical threshold is high.

Favorable fitness activities: rock climbing, weight training, bodybuilding, step aerobics, spinning, step machine, rowing, mountain biking, running, soccer, hockey, aerobic boxing, calisthenics, military-type workouts.

Type IV. The Creative Idealist: EIFP, EIFJ, IIFP, IIFJ

It's important for you to feel self-fulfilled, and you're not apt to follow trends. You're fine either training at home alone or doing your thing at the gym. Your threshold for physical stress is high, and you like exercise that's intense. You usually don't have much trouble finding new ways to enjoy working out.

Favorable fitness activities: mountain biking, aerobics (all types), active team sports, weight training, bodybuilding, cross-training, freestyle dance.

Genetic Limitations: Fit into Your Fitness Genes

People with lean or muscular genes should appreciate that it's a gift. It's a gift that not many people have, despite what our culture implies. For those who find it a cinch to get fit, who've never battled the bulge, it's hard to imagine that so many people are struggling to reach their goals. Most of us, though, must accept the fact that we can't always get what we want, no matter how hard we push ourselves or how many things we do right. While parts of our bodies are apt to respond very well to the way we train, other parts, despite what we do, will be far more resistant to change. I don't make this point to discourage you or to make you feel worse than you do. Instead, it's my way of *encouraging* you to reframe how you look at your "flaws," to urge you to start making more of the best and to start making less of the worst.

If you tend to be idealistic (or optimistic, if you prefer), to hear that your genes may be limiting you may be difficult to accept. But if parts of your body are predisposed to be diet or workout resistant, busting your hump in the face of this fact just underscores that it's a fact! The point here is that the effort you're making to alter your personal "flaws" might be better spent in a different way instead of combating your genes. If you've spent many months, or years, in the gym, obsessed with correcting your faults, it's important to see that your only real fault was to think that your actions were wise.

Okay, you say, so my genes present some challenges others don't have. How do I learn to accept myself and to be less obsessed with my flaws? What options do I have left to me now, if there really are things I can't change? Consider the following thoughts about possible ways to address your concerns.

Top Four Ways to Accept or Thwart Your Body Type Limitations

1. *Practice self-acceptance.* To achieve, maintain, and reinforce unconditional self-acceptance, contact a thought-field therapist, or learn more about TFT. It will help you to view your body in a much more forgiving way.

2. *Learn to change your perspective with regard to what's good and bad; learn to see the upside of some of the things that are getting you down.* Learn new ways to appreciate different things about how you look. For example, instead of viewing your calves as scrawny or pitifully small, see them instead as "sprinter's calves"—lean, well toned, and defined. Or see a bulge as a "sensuous curve" or a "built-in flotation device." Okay, I admit it's a bit of a stretch, but it's just so you get the point. Look for what's good instead of what's bad; focus on strengths and not flaws. It'll help you to change your perspective about yourself and the way you work out.

3. *Reframe your view of the variables that determine your physical fate.* Sometimes, getting in shape can be a remarkably humbling task. You may, for example, when taking a class, doing leg lifts to tone up your tush, wonder why Barbie's twin sister seems to be toning up hers twice as fast. Meanwhile, she's probably looking at you and thinking the very same thing. You want her butt, she wants your arms, and you both want each other's legs. Too often, the things you yearn for most are the things that you don't (or can't) have.

   There are many genetic factors that determine your fitness fate. While your fiber-type ratio and body type must be factored into the mix, you must also consider the points where your muscles insert relative to your joints. Add to the list kinesthetic sense (the "feel" you have for a movement), and it's easy to see how improving your strength can be more complex than you think.

   Putting this into perspective allows for a healthier frame of mind. It lessens our impulse to beat ourselves up when we fall a bit short of our goals. It helps us to see how, sometimes, what we achieve is beyond our control. For example, the point where your muscles insert in relation to bones and joints determines the level of strength you have with respect to the way you move. To illustrate, while your biceps muscle originates at the shoulder, the insertion point is the radius (a bone in your lower arm). So if you're performing a biceps curl, and your biceps inserts *near* the joint, you're likely to find it hard to perform this movement with lots of weight. Conversely, if your insertion point is farther away from the joint, all other things being equal, you'll be able to lift more weight. Whenever this point is close to a joint, you're mechanically "disadvantaged." Imagine that you've grasped a fishing rod with your hands very close together. If you try to pull in a fish this way, it's going to be hard to do. The farther apart your hands are, though, the lighter the fish will be. All things being equal, when it comes to lifting a weight, the person who has better "leverage" is the one who has greater strength.

4. *If you have a healthy self-image, and your expectations are sound, consider a surgical "cure" (if the option you choose has a very low risk).* To consider going the surgical route for your workout-resistant problems, each of the following questions should elicit a yes response.

◆ EXERCISE ◆

Is Cosmetic (Plastic) Surgery an Option You Should Consider?

Put an X next to each statement that directly applies to you.

—— I've shared my concerns with a therapist who's familiar with image disorders and agrees that my choice to have surgery is for reasons that truly make sense.

—— I can honestly say that I've done all I can to improve "problem" parts of my body, but the results I've achieved are minimal and fail to reflect my efforts.

—— I've consulted with two or more surgeons, and I've seen the results of their work. All are board-certified doctors who are experienced in their field.

——— I've learned all I can about all of the facts that concern me and my procedure. I'm abreast of the latest advances, and I've made a well-informed choice. (For example, today liposuction is much safer and more effective, allowing for far less blood loss and a more even removal of fat.)

——— My doctor has ruled out problems that present a surgical risk.

——— I don't *need* to have this procedure performed, but it's something I'd *like* to do.

——— I accept my body the way it is, despite my limitations.

——— My expectations are reasonable; perfection is not my goal. I'd like to improve my proportions, be less self-conscious, and wear new clothes, but I don't hope to have a perfect result, only a change for the better.

——— My body is fit and fairly well toned; my skin is youthful and taut.

——— Changing my body is *my* choice alone; it's not to please anyone else.

◆ ◆ ◆

Cosmetic surgery can make sense only *if* it involves little risk. For a small number of my clients, it was a choice they were glad that they made. All of them, though, were fit, self-assured, well-informed, and in excellent health. Their decision was made after long, hard thought and only when all else failed. While procedures like breast augmentation tend to involve a much greater risk, no one but *you* can decide how the pros add up and compare to the cons. Just make sure you're objective and fully aware of what the cons are. Don't make an impulsive decision that someday you might regret.

Why are these all important things to keep in the back of your mind? Because if you're getting down on yourself for something you think you lack, there could be factors beyond your control that are limiting your success. Remembering this may help you to be less concerned about how you compare. The truth is that it's all relative—we all have our own unique strengths.

Heredity sets limits, environment decides the exact portion within these limits.

—EDWIN CARLTON MCDOWELL

Nutritional UFOs

The Things We Don't Know That Hurt Us

*Give me a dozen heartbreaks, if it helps me to lose
a few pounds.*

—Colette

It seems as if more and more experts these days are professing
that diets don't work. Because diets are often hazardous to our
mental and physical health, they say that the chances they'll work for us
are, in general, slim to none. I believe this is true, to a point. I agree
that diets, when viewed on the whole, cause people more harm than
good, but often it's not the diet that's wrong, it's the context in which it
is followed. In fact, I'm convinced that the crux of the problem basically
comes down to this: Diets don't work because *people* don't work on the
things that would make diets work! You might want to read that last line
again—it makes an important point. It's not the type of diet you're on
that is truly the key to success. Instead it's how willing and able you are
to change your attachment to food. To do this, you must learn to address
your nutritional UFOs.

This chapter examines obstacles to achieving nutritional health. It
exposes the misconceptions that are most apt to get you off track and
helps you to recognize hidden ways that you may undermine your success. By citing the top ten UFOs that make diet goals hard to reach,
this chapter helps you identify those that are likely to hinder *you* most.

In the same way that people think "working out right" is the essence of getting in shape, most people also think "dieting right" is the secret to taking off weight. It's this kind of misguided viewpoint that sets most dieters up to fail. Although it's important to eat in a way that is safe and nutritionally sound, it's exposing your personal obstacles that is truly the key to success. If you don't do this, you'll be constantly foiled by the same exact UFOs. Until you learn how to put yourself in the right frame of body and mind, no matter how good your diet may be the outcome will be the same. You'll lose a few pounds, regain what you've lost, and find yourself back at square one.

To understand my perspective on this, consider Cindy's story. "I have to admit," said Cindy, "that I'm powerless over food. No matter how hard I exercise, or what kind of diet I try, I'm lucky to lose any weight at all—in fact, I usually don't! I need a diet that helps me to lose a lot of weight really fast. Give me the one that they put Oprah on—let's see if it works for me!"

"The diet that's best for you, Cindy," I said, "is the one that accounts for *your* needs. No one diet is always best, or right, for each single person. It's also important for you to know that a diet will never work if you fail to take steps to identify and conquer your UFOs. Once we reveal and remove the blocks that are likely to get in your way, then we can talk about how to decide the best way for you to eat."

As it turned out, Cindy was diagnosed to have ADD (attention deficit disorder). In addition, based on the things she said (and the things about her I observed), it was clear to me that her ADD was her primary UFO. Because she had trouble focusing and following through on most tasks, Cindy had never been able to stay on a diet for more than three days. Because she was always so scattered and going at such a frenetic pace, she found it a chore to prepare and buy food, let alone make healthy food choices.

When Cindy was treated for ADD, all of this started to change. As she found herself starting to focus more on the things that would serve her best, she made it a point to start taking more time to plan and prepare healthy meals. She also stopped feeling so out of control with regard to the things that she craved. Moreover, she started to exercise more, as often as six times a week.

Now that Cindy was feeling a lot more focused and self-assured, I provided her with a diet to help her accomplish her weight-loss goal. But although she did find it helpful, and actually lost about five or six pounds, she had an additional UFO that still hadn't been addressed. When Cindy confessed that she often craved things like cereal, pasta, and bread, she gave me a clue about what it could be that continued to get in her way. Because her body was sensitive to high-carbohydrate foods, she found that when eating a lot of them, she couldn't lose any more weight. But once she varied her diet (to include more high-protein foods), it served to rev up her metabolism and helped her to burn more fat. The pounds then began dropping off again, and Cindy was right back on track.

By this time, Cindy had lost fifteen pounds and had only ten more to go. But once again, something came to the fore that proceeded to get in her way. Because in the past she'd been deeply hurt by a man she used to date, as she closed in on her weight-loss goal, it brought up some long-standing fears. She feared that if she achieved her goal, and started to date once again, it would mean that she'd have to risk getting hurt in the same way she was in the past. This was an issue that Cindy resolved through the use of TFT. Once we peeled back the layers, exposing her anger, suspicion, and fear, we freed up all of the energy blocks that she held with regard to her past. Once she stopped fearing relationships, and let go of her negative thoughts, she promptly began to lose more weight and easily reached her goal.

This should give you a pretty good sense of the way the process unfolds. While at times exposing and learning to thwart a single block suffices, more often you'll find that a number of things are nutritional UFOs. It's peeling the layers back, one by one, that gets you where you want to be. Once you catch onto the process, it's not quite as hard as it seems.

Top Ten Nutritional UFOs

1. A "ONE-DIET-FITS-ALL" WAY OF THINKING

Too many people hold the belief that there's one route to weight-loss success, that "one perfect diet" exists, somewhere, that will help them to reach their goals. They remind me, at times, of miners sifting through diets as if they were gold, or of pirates hunting for treasure, who think that the diet is some sort of "map." If you tend to view diets this way too, then you might want to ask yourself this: If your diet sage claims that it's he or she who has found the only right map, then why do so few of their followers ever get to the spot marked "X"? It's thinking this way, believing in maps, that sets people up to fail. While the map may well be a good one, and may point in the right direction, if it's not one you're able to follow and read, it'll do you no good at all.

The point here is that finding the right type of diet is only one step, one small overemphasized part of what you must do to succeed. Because people fail to appreciate this and focus so much on "the diet," whenever they start falling short of their goals, it's the diet that gets all the blame. This is like blaming the personal ads when the people you're meeting are jerks! People don't own the part *they* play with regard to where they end up. Moreover, they don't look at variables that are critical to their success.

◆ EXERCISE ◆

Have Nutritional UFOs Kept You from Achieving Your Physical Goals?

Put an X next to each statement that directly applies to you.

—— I often have very strong cravings that I haven't been able to curb.

—— Dairy foods don't agree with me. They make me feel bloated and full.

—— I'm currently taking drugs that affect my appetite or my mood (anti-depressant drugs that have increased my desire to eat, or antihypertensive drugs that caused me to feel depressed).

—— It's possible that I'm allergic to foods that are processed or made with yeast (cereal, pastry, bread, pasta, cookies, crackers, and cakes).

—— My blood sugar is unstable after consuming carb-laden foods.

—— I've noticed that my emotions are linked to my cravings for certain foods.

—— I often have indigestion, constipation, heartburn, or gas.

—— I crave certain foods when premenstrual.

—— More often than not, I feel depressed. My mood affects how I eat.

◆ ◆ ◆

In other words, what are the UFOs that are most apt to be in your way? If any one of these questions has evoked a yes response, the odds are good that *no* diet will work—until you address your concerns. Now, can you see how losing weight involves more than meets the eye? For those who are dealing with problems involving their image, their body, or food, these problems have to be treated in very specific, personal ways. One's pattern of intake, supplementation, and foods emphasized (or avoided) must be carefully individualized for a diet to actually work.

2. UNHEALTHY, NARROW PERCEPTIONS OF WHAT THE WORD *DIETING* REALLY MEANS

Most people don't see dieting as a long-term, continuing process. Instead, it's viewed as a one-time, go-for-broke, fixed, time-limited goal. For example, a bride, to look svelte in her dress, goes on a "prenuptial fast," or, for a class reunion, people crash diet the week before. You don't need me to remind you that this isn't a good thing to do. Regardless, I'm guessing that you, like me, have done things like this before.

Maybe it's the word "diet" that gives us such a shortsighted view. The phrase "to go on a diet" implies restricting your intake of food, adhering to some rigid regimen that will help you to lose lots of weight. It also implies that the diet is at some point going to end, creating the notion that then you'll go back to a more "normal" way to eat. This just creates a mind-set that is setting you up to fail.

I have a little suggestion that may help to reframe your view. Let's replace the term "diet" with one that resonates more with good health. A healthy "nutritional plan" implies that you'll make a more permanent change. It doesn't imply strict adherence to something that's hard or unpleasant to do, and it doesn't have connotations implying that what you will do is short-lived. Instead, it means doing whatever you must to achieve and maintain better health. By learning to shift your perspective of what the word dieting really means, you'll not only see diets differently, you'll see yourself differently too.

3. INAPPROPRIATE BALANCE OF CARBOHYDRATES, PROTEIN, AND FAT

If you're reading this book, there's a pretty good chance that you've read a few diet books too. And like most people are these days, you're probably very confused. Who wouldn't be, with so many new and contrasting points of view? For example, while some are convinced that it's carbohydrates we need to curb, others contend that carbs are the core of a healthy, well-balanced diet. Some say do it one way, others say do it another. Who should we put our faith in, and how can we tell what works best? How can we know which diet will help us the most to achieve our goals?

The truth is that we're all different and have different things in our way. The type of diet we follow must account for our personal needs. For example, a diet that's low in fat and high in complex carbs may work very well for some folks but may not be what's right for you. To illustrate, if you tend to crave carbs, and your body is insulin-sensitive, this kind of diet could keep you from reaching your health and nutritional goals. Because overdoing the carbs will cause your insulin levels to spike, your blood sugar won't remain stable enough for your energy level to last. This will limit your energy, strength, and endurance whenever you train. Moreover, if you're like most folks, and you truly are insulin-sensitive, a carb-laden diet is actually apt to prevent you from burning fat. Because when your insulin level is high, your "fat-burning furnace" cools down, a signal gets sent to your body to start burning fat at a much slower rate. This signal comes from eicosanoids (your hormones for hormone control). When an overproduction of insulin creates eicosanoids that are "bad," they prevent your body from breaking down fat in the areas where it is stored. This is the crux of the argument used to support diet plans like the Zone, which are based on the theory that generally it is the carbs that are making us fat.

Although they still have some bugs to work out, and to some are still controversial, modern-day diets (such as the Zone) have at least put us on the right track. Insulin-sensitivity is very clearly a widespread problem. If you're wondering why I'm so sure of this, it's because I believe what I see. Attesting to what Barry Sears reports in his popular book *The Zone*, three-quarters of all of my clients haven't lost weight any other way. Seventy-five percent report that they crave lots of starchy foods and notice dramatic energy swings that relate to the things that they eat. For the others, a higher-carb diet makes better sense, if it's what they prefer. Sixty percent of their diet is normally made up of complex carbs, while their protein percentage is 20 percent, the same as it is for fat. Conversely, plans like the Zone that encourage a diet involving less carbs suggest that one's daily carb intake should be no more than 40 percent (the protein percentage is 30 percent, the same as it is for fat). This specific balance of substrates (carbohydrates, protein, and fat) is suggested for insulin-sensitive folks, if possible, at every meal. The sources of carbs that are favored are those with the *lowest glycemic index*, a term that refers to the rate at which carbohydrates enter the blood. The lower the glycemic index, the slower the rate of absorption. The slower the rate of absorption, the better your body burns fat.

Foods with a Low Glycemic Index*
Fructose
Barley
Pears
Peas
Lentils
Grapefruit
Cherries
Plums
Apples
Apple juice
Grapes
Peaches
Oatmeal (slow-cooking)
Kidney beans
Chickpeas
Lima beans
Tomato soup

Yogurt
Whole-grain rye bread

*Good, if you're insulin-sensitive

Foods with a High Glycemic Index*
Puffed rice
Rice cakes
Most cereals
Puffed wheat
Instant rice
Foods containing simple sugars (such as maltose and glucose)
White or whole-wheat bread
Oat bran
Instant mashed potatoes
White and brown rice
Carrots
Corn
Bananas
Raisins
Low-fat ice cream
Corn chips
Pasta

*Bad, if you're insulin-sensitive

When you follow a Zone-type diet, you focus on eating "good" (monounsaturated) fat. Good fat gets rid of the kind of bad fat that is hazardous to your health. Popular sources of good fat include canola oil and olives, as well as macadamia nuts, avocados, and olive oil. The gist of a balanced Zone diet consists, by and large, of *protein* and *produce*—mostly lean sources of protein, "healthy fat," fresh veggies, and fruit. By restricting yourself to these types of food, even though you're consuming more fat, the balance is such that your body burns what you consume in a much better way.

How do you know that you're getting the balance of substrates that you require? Dr. Sears recommends that you learn to think of your food in terms of "blocks." For example, one piece of fruit is roughly considered two blocks of carbs. In his book, he provides guidelines for converting your food into blocks and suggests that you measure these blocks by making each portion the size of your palm. Although I have some clients who say that this guideline works quite well, others don't seem to trust it and prefer to be more precise. For them, I suggest a "diet coach," to assist them in tracking their meals. The diet coach (see the Appendix) is a computer that fits in your hand, much like those used as daytimers or to translate a foreign language. Specialty product catalogs like Sharper Image or Inner Balance often feature items like this at a fairly reasonable cost. The diet coach keeps a running tab of everything you consume and can break it down into percentages of carbohydrates, protein, and fat. This way, you know exactly whether or not you are in "the Zone." Moreover, once you develop a sense for what combinations are best, you won't have to use the computer as much, except when you try something new.

Although the Zone plan is a good one, and has worked well for most of my clients, I've found that it has a few shortcomings that are not very often addressed. First, a Zone-type diet doesn't allow for a whole lot of food, at least not in terms of calories, or compared to a typical diet. Dr. Sears addresses this point by claiming that when "in the Zone," your cravings are apt to be less severe and you're likely to *want* less food. I've found this is not always true, though—the cravings don't always subside. Those who are insulin-sensitive often crave high-glycemic foods, and generally staying away from them is a difficult thing to do. Although it's important to highlight the value of putting a limit on carbs, asking carb addicts to eat fewer carbs is like saying to smokers, *Don't smoke!* The reasons that people have food cravings aren't only physiologic. They have to do with emotional blocks and energy blocks as well. The best way I've found to release these blocks is, again, through TFT. By using Zone guidelines, with TFT, my clients have had great success.

The Zone approach also doesn't account for unsuitable food combinations. For example, some experts claim that vegetables shouldn't be eaten with fruit, as our body requires different enzymes to fully digest different types of foods. While many reject the notion that food combinations are much of a factor, I've found that for some of my clients there's no question at all that it is. When this is the case, and I have a client who also is insulin-sensitive, I have them adjust how they eat in a way that accounts for both these concerns. By using a food log or journal, and allowing for some trial and error, we focus our efforts to glean an approach that accounts for their personal needs.

While critics of Zone-type diets claim that the science behind them is weak, proponents claim just the opposite: that the research is tried-and-true. If you're in a quandary about whom to trust and about what will serve you best, what I suggest is that, first, you abandon all notions of having blind faith. Then you can do what I've learned to do—trust what *you* find works the best. This may sound like a trite thing to say, but I don't know of many who do! Instead, they get swayed by the latest new trend and keep finding themselves more confused. Do what makes the most sense *for you* first, then give it some time to work. Then, if it doesn't, before you give up, find out if you have other blocks. Before you start blaming your diet plan for your failure to reach your goals, make sure that additional UFOs aren't making the right plan *wrong*.

◆ **EXERCISE** ◆

Is Insulin-Sensitivity a Nutritional UFO?

Put an X next to each statement that directly applies to you.

—— I tend to crave high-glycemic foods (such as cereal, bread, white rice, carrots, corn, bananas, raisins, corn chips, candy, pasta, and pretzels).

—— I have frequent, significant energy swings that I notice more after I eat.

—— When I take performance-enhancing drinks or consume "high-energy" bars, it gives me a boost for a very short time, but then I feel very fatigued.

—— I feel foggy, light-headed, dizzy, or "spaced" when I go for too long without carbs.

—— I often wake up with "carb hangovers" (after eating high-carb evening meals).

Scoring
The more of these statements you've marked with an X, the more you are insulin-sensitive. A diet that has the proper balance of protein, fat, and

carbs is essential for you to burn more fat and improve your overall health (30 percent protein, 30 percent fat, 40 percent carbohydrates).

◆ ◆ ◆

4. FOOD ALLERGIES/INTOLERANCES

Food allergies and intolerances are more common than most people think. Because so much of the food we eat contains chemicals, hormones, and dyes, the odds that these foods will be toxic to us are better than you might guess. Wheat and yeast are the most common foods to which many of us are allergic, as are sugar and dairy products, such as cereal, milk, and eggs. Mushrooms, coffee, corn, and fruit can be problematic as well, but by no means are they the only foods that could cause an allergic response. Enzyme-depleted, chemically altered, highly processed food can seldom be put in our body without there being some price to pay.

Consuming these types of foods is like filling a gas tank with dirty fuel. Often they rob us of enzymes we need to digest and assimilate food. When this occurs consistently, we develop a food intolerance.

Food allergies are different. Whenever the food we fail to digest is perceived by our body as toxic, our white blood cells overcompensate and cause an allergic response. Often this type of response becomes more apparent over time.

The truth is that many nutritionists fail to take this into account. Food allergies and intolerances can be prominent UFOs. If your diet includes particular foods that you have a hard time breaking down, your body must use lots of energy to clean up what you don't digest. And if you have an allergic response to a food that you often consume, you'll feel so drained and fatigued that you probably won't have the strength to work out. Headaches and gastrointestinal ills are common allergic responses, as are indigestion, rapid pulse, and marked fatigue. If these are symptoms you typically have when consuming particular foods, until you begin to abstain from them, you'll struggle to lose any weight.

How do you know if you really do have a food allergy or an intolerance? While allergy tests can help you gauge your reaction to different foods, there are two very simple procedures that you can use to see where you stand.

Muscle Testing for Food Allergies/Intolerances

1. *Hold one arm out straight to the side and parallel to the floor.*
2. *Have someone place a hand on your lower arm or around your wrist.*
3. *In the hand of your opposite arm, hold the item you wish to test.*
4. *Place the item you're testing flush against either of these locations:* against your diaphragm, which is located under your breastbone, or against your thyroid, which is between your collarbones. (Note: The substance you're testing can be in or out of its package.)
5. *Attempt to raise your straight arm up against your partner's hand.* He or she should try to push down while you are resisting their effort.
6. *If you're testing strong (your partner finds that your arm is hard to force down), you're* not *apt to be allergic to the substance you hold in your hand.* If you're testing weak (your partner is easily able to force your arm down), you *are* apt to be allergic to the substance you hold in your hand.

Coca's Pulse Test for Food Allergies

1. *Take your pulse before you consume the food that you wish to test.* Record the result.
2. *Maintain a relaxed position in a place where you don't feel stressed.*
3. *Wait fifteen or twenty minutes and then take your pulse again.* If your heart rate is ten beats higher (or more), you're likely to have a food allergy.

I'm often amazed by how accurate these types of tests turn out to be. In particular, it's always fun for me to muscle-test foods with my clients. It's the stupefied look on their faces that amuses me most of all. Most find it hard to imagine that they're so allergic to certain foods. They also find it hard to believe that these foods can limit their strength. It's not just their strength that's affected, though, it's their energy level as well. Whether they find it hard to work out, or hard to succeed on a diet, food allergies or intolerances are their primary UFOs.

Top Ten Ways to Overcome a Food Allergy or Intolerance

1. *Ask your physician about high-fiber or colon-cleansing supplements*. Using these types of supplements slows the absorption of problem-prone food.

2. *Remember not to take aspirin within three hours of any meal*. A British medical journal study reports that when aspirin is used, a greater amount of an allergy-causing food is often absorbed.

3. *Periodically, go on a cleanse*. Try to avoid all allergy-causing foods for sixty days. Then, if you like, you can reintroduce them gradually into your diet. It's possible, though, that after your cleanse, because you feel so much better, you'll decide to abstain from the foods you gave up (that caused an allergic response). You should notice, as well, that your cravings are quelled or significantly reduced.

4. *If you have any question about which foods are actually giving you trouble, in general avoid the following:* bananas, beef, caffeine, chocolate, citrus fruit, corn, dairy products, eggs, oats, oysters, peanuts, salmon, strawberries, tomatoes, wheat, white rice, yeast, and all processed/refined food products. These are the foods most likely to cause a problem for sensitive people. It'll help you to make a list of the top ten foods you crave the most (the things we are most allergic to are often the things we most crave). By avoiding these foods every now and then, you can curb your allergic response.

5. *Examine the labels of packaged foods to determine the presence of dyes*. F, D, and C (#5 yellow) dyes should consistently be avoided. Also avoid vanillin, benzyldehyde, eucalyptol, monosodium glutamate (MSG), BHT-BHA, benzoates, and annatto.

6. *Vary your cycle of foods*. People who have food allergies often rotate the foods that they eat. No one food is ever consumed for more than four days in succession, and then at least four days must pass before eating that food again. This prevents your white blood cells from trying to fight disagreeable foods. Cycling your foods is often enough to prevent an allergic response.

7. *Avoid foods containing sulfites (if you're sensitive to this substance)*. This includes avocados, carrots, mushrooms, peppers,

tomatoes, potatoes, most shellfish, pickles, potato chips, dry-mix salad dressings, canned soups, beer, cider, fruit juice, gelatin, and wine. Check all labels carefully when purchasing packaged foods.

8. *Take hypoallergenic supplements.* Make sure, before purchasing supplements, that they don't include common allergens. Review all labels thoroughly and compare before making a purchase.

9. *Consult a holistic practitioner (herbalist, naturopath, homeopath, allergist, nutritionist) for advice about using herbs.* Those often recommended include: burdock, centaury, dandelion, fringe tree, phytolacca, and St. Mary's Thistle. While some herbs can help with food allergies, others can minimize cravings. To eliminate your food cravings, or at least to keep them at bay, it would benefit you to contact those well-trained in TFT. (To contact a thought-field therapist, refer to the Appendix.)

10. *Use these acupressure points to relieve and to overcome symptoms. Three Mile Point*: four finger widths below the knee, on the outside part of the leg; *Outer Gate*: two and one-half finger widths above the crease in the wrist, between the ulna and radius bones of the forearm (on the top); *Sea of Energy*: directly under the navel, two finger widths below; *Elegant Mansion*: in the hollow below the collarbone on either side of the sternum. Using these points either one at a time or together in combination can help you to overcome symptoms related to allergy-causing foods. Hold each point for a minute (or more) and repeat until symptoms subside.

Meridian Point to Curb Cravings for Allergy-Causing Foods

Four Whites: Directly under either eye (on the facial bone indentation). If you move your finger around, you'll feel exactly where this point is. Press or tap the four whites spot while thinking about what you crave. Repeat as often as needed until your craving subsides.

5. IMPROPER FOOD COMBINING

If you've ever read *Fit for Life* by researchers Harvey and Marilyn Diamond, some of the things I'll be telling you here are things you've already heard. While compared to most diet gurus they have unconventional views, the Diamonds have raised some points that may be important to bear in mind. Their advice with regard to combining foods in essence boils down to this: Because different types of food require different enzymes to be digested, there are certain combinations that you shouldn't eat at the same time. For example, they say fruits and vegetables should never be eaten together, as your body breaks down and absorbs these foods in uniquely different ways. In addition, they claim that fruit is the ideal choice to start your day, as it's broken down fairly easily and provides the best "energy fuel" (this is in contrast to Zone-like plans, which suggest, if you're insulin-sensitive, that it's best to include some protein and fat for fuel that burns slower and lasts). They also advise eating vegetables once the fruit has had time to digest. Potatoes, dairy, meat, and grains (believed to be less healthy options) are said to be best later on in the day, when your body requires less fuel. By consuming fruits and vegetables when you're more active (during the day), they claim that you'll have more energy and improve your overall health.

Basic Food-Combining Rules
◆ Never eat fruits with vegetables.
◆ Never eat protein with starch.
◆ If possible, eat the following foods, in this order, throughout the day: fruits; vegetables; nuts and seeds; grains, breads, and potatoes; chicken, fish, and red meat; dairy products.
◆ Combine as few different foods as you can at each individual meal.

Michael's "More Practical" Food-Combining Rules
◆ Never eat fruits with vegetables. (If you do, have some Maalox at hand.)
◆ Try not to eat any protein with starch, for example, chicken with pasta. If you do, take digestive enzymes just before you consume your meal.

- ◆ Choose foods from the meat, grain, and dairy groups during the latter half of your day.
- ◆ While maintaining an optimum substrate balance (like the Zone, if you're insulin-sensitive), combine as few different foods as you can for each individual meal.
- ◆ When protein-rich foods are combined with foods that are higher in carbs or fat, always consume higher-protein foods first, to facilitate good digestion.

While the Diamonds' advice is compelling and in many ways does make sense, eating like this is difficult if you're trying to stay "in the Zone." If you truly are insulin-sensitive, and you eat only fruit at one meal, your insulin levels are likely to rise very quickly and then quickly fall. According to fans of nutritional plans that encourage a Zone-like balance, this results in less energy and a slower metabolic rate. If it's true that three out of four of us are actually insulin-sensitive, this would make the *Fit for Life* plan poorly suited for people in general. But if you're *not* insulin-sensitive, it's something you should bear in mind. Improper food combinations may be acting as UFOs.

Personally, I find it hard to stay in the Zone with the *Fit for Life* plan. But as much as is practical, I watch how my foods are combined. For example, I never eat veggies with fruit, but I do eat veggies with fish. Or, when I'm having a salad, I eat nuts to add protein and fat. This serves not only to help me maintain an effective Zone-type balance but also to let me eat in a way that supports my digestive health. In short, I do the best I can to integrate both approaches, without ever being obsessed about strictly adhering to either plan. If I feel that my energy level has waned, I look at what I've been eating. Then, I refrain from combining some foods to see if I notice a change. My advice is that you try doing the same and then write down how you feel. By keeping a food log or diary, you can find out what serves you best. If you think that you're insulin-sensitive and are combining the wrong types of foods, try both approaches for two or three days to find out what works best for you. This should help you to be more clear about what's going to help you most.

6. MISUNDERSTANDING THE VALUE AND ROLE OF COMMON NUTRITIONAL SUPPLEMENTS

This is one of those subjects that makes me want to pull out my hair. So many inane, spurious claims are made about supplementation that it's almost an insurmountable task to glean all the facts from the fibs. While supplements certainly can help—when used in the right kind of way—the way they are normally used and prescribed is rarely, if ever, correct. Not only that, but too many times they hurt a lot more than they help! To understand why this is the case, consider the following facts.

Supplement "experts" fail to account for our vast, biochemical differences. The way we digest and metabolize food varies from person to person, but often when we take supplements we fail to acknowledge this fact. Supplements aren't like aspirin; there isn't one dose that works best. Some need more, some need less, and some don't need them at all. For example, a ninety-pound woman who is frail and very small-boned may need more of a certain vitamin than does a two-hundred-fifty-pound man. Moreover, when they're combined, or used in conjunction with certain drugs, supplements don't always work in the same, predictable, straightforward way. When some people take a whole lot of different supplements all at one time, their benefits are neutralized, they cancel each other out. While most people *can* derive benefit from taking several at the same time, other folks require far less, as too many spoil the brew.

The challenge with taking supplements lies in the dose and the type one takes. It's also important to have an idea about how they are best combined. Because most recommendations are simply guesses about what's best, the way that most people take supplements tends to be woefully imprecise. In addition, we're much too trusting. We accept all the claims, believe all the hype, and fail to examine all sides. Perhaps instead of being so quick to accept all the things we hear, we should first make an effort to flush out the facts and examine the pros and the cons. For example, the supplement creatine has received widespread acclaim. Creatine, a unique combination of certain amino acids, is used for developing muscle mass or increasing endurance and strength. While many swear by creatine and believe that it really does help, it's possible that if *you* take it, it will do you more harm than good. Creatine functions to help muscle fibers use more ATP (ATP is the energy source that fuels and supports your cells). For creatine to be utilized effectively in your body, it is best combined with glucose, which helps creatine enter your cells. But although when taking creatine, glucose aids in its absorption, for those who are insulin-sensitive, this may not be a good thing. Because the addition of glucose can cause insulin levels to spike, these levels could drop dramatically within a fairly short span of time. I've tried creatine a few times myself, and what happens is always the same: I get a quick boost of energy, then, before very long, I crash. If you're clearly not insulin-sensitive, creatine may work fine. But be certain to do your homework before you decide to give it a try.

Most people don't take their supplements the right way or at the right time. When people gulp down powders and pills, it's often at inopportune times. Some supplements, for example, work best when your stomach is empty. Others are more effective when they're taken with some type of food. It can't just be any food, though; the food must be "supplement-friendly." Let's say that you're lactose intolerant, and you mix protein powder with milk. Because your digestion will suffer, much of the protein won't be absorbed, and as a result it's likely that most of the nutrients will go to waste. Though supplement manufacturers offer advice about taking their products, you need to find out what works best for *you* (biochemically, we're all unique). You may want to see a nutritionist or a naturopathic physician to determine the best way to utilize and to combine whatever you take.

At this point, you may be inclined to think, "It's more complex than I thought. I guess that there's really no sure-fire way to know what I really need." This isn't exactly true. The least you can do is improve your odds that your supplements really will work. Here's what I suggest you do to determine what's best for you.

1. *See a naturopath or homeopath for a personalized prescription.* Don't just guess about what you need; let an expert help you find out. Whether they test your blood, saliva, urine, or samples of hair, different doctors use different tests to determine your personal needs. I know of one doctor who uses a test that works especially well. By means of a process some people call a "biodermal assay," he measures how parts of the body respond to each

supplement type he tests. By placing a wand or "sensor" against the meridian points on your hand, he can make a precise assessment of your unique nutritional needs. He can tell what you should and shouldn't use and the best supplement combinations. I've sent quite a few of my clients his way, and they've all had outstanding results. Even though some people scoff at the way this doctor conducts his tests, when it comes to deciding on supplements, it sure beats making a guess. There are many holistic practitioners who can fine-tune your supplement needs, so it may be worth your while to find an experienced one near you.

2. *Experiment with some muscle tests to determine your supplement needs.* You can use the food allergy muscle test (see page 159) for your supplement needs as well. By holding the supplement(s) you want to test on your thyroid or diaphragm, you can work with a partner to get an idea about what types will work for you best. You can also test combinations of things to see which work well together. This test works best to determine what's *not* apt to work as opposed to what will. Although it isn't a perfect test, and should not be implicitly trusted, with patience and perseverance you can usually get good results.

The day will come when people will spend their whole lives on a diet modeled for their specific genetic pattern.
—DR. DARLA DANFORD, NATIONAL INSTITUTES OF HEALTH

7. DIET FOODS OFTEN AREN'T HEALTHY AND MAY NOT EVEN BE LOW-CALORIE

Many foods that are touted to be dietetic, low-fat, or low-cal contain less calories only because they in fact contain less food. You're unlikely to feel very satisfied eating prepackaged, low-calorie meals. They may appear appetizing, but they're rarely what you expect.

In addition, these meals more often than not contain high levels of salt, not to mention preservatives, chemical additives, and/or dyes. It's important to be more scrupulous when you go shopping for "diet" foods. Read all labels carefully and be conscious about what they say. Remember, for some types of diet foods, low-fat isn't really low-fat. They may have *less* fat, but only compared to another similar choice.

8. INEFFICIENT FOOD DISTRIBUTION; CONSUMING HEAVY, HIGH-CALORIE MEALS TWO TO THREE TIMES A DAY

Although this is no revelation, perhaps you could use a reminder: You make more efficient use of your fuel if you don't always top off your tank. Instead of filling it up to the brim every time you stop at the station, leave your tank a bit empty and select a better-grade fuel. Your body, besides running cleaner (and without such a noisy exhaust), will feel a lot lighter and less bogged down with the stuff that you don't burn off.

To spare you any more metaphors, it basically works like this: If you eat more food than your body needs, you store what you don't need as fat. Or the part that you don't store ends up being turned into waste. When you eat smaller meals more consistently, your metabolism stays stoked. You burn more calories and more fat and feel better while you do. You're also less prone to have blood-sugar swings and less apt to crave the wrong foods.

This is a pattern of eating that, when practical, makes good sense. The problem that most people have with it is learning to plan ahead. Some people choose one day to precook all the food that they need for a week (premeasured portions are frozen to be consumed whenever desired). Because they've preprepared their food for small meals throughout the day, they less often choose the wrong kinds of foods, especially when they are bored. When the right food is there when you need it, you're less apt to reach for what's wrong.

9. FREQUENT EXPOSURE TO FATTENING OR UNHEALTHY CHOICES OF FOOD

If you often attend business lunches, parties, or business-related functions, your risk is high when it comes to being tempted by fattening foods. In addition, if family gatherings often involve sharing lavish meals, you're also more likely to find that it's hard to eat in a clean, healthy way.

If you can't avoid situations that expose you to fattening foods, perhaps you can learn to change the way you prepare, react, and respond. Here's what I suggest you do, if you find that this is the case.

- *Before you attend a function, always have something to eat.* This will help you to stay in control when surrounded by fattening foods. When you show up hungry (or anxious), you put yourself more at risk.
- *Fill up on healthy foods first.* Veggies or watered-down juices are your smartest and safest bet, but never consume them together because they're digested in different ways. Never stand or sit near foods that you tend to pick at or crave.
- *Use this acupressure point to eliminate nervous hunger.* The *Grand Luo* point is four finger widths below the pit of your arm. Holding this point for a minute or more is apt to help calm your nerves.
- *Use this acupressure point to reduce or eliminate cravings.* The point *Four Whites* is under each eye on the facial bone indentation.
- *Take a high-fiber supplement to curb your appetite during the day.* Not only do high-fiber supplements help you feel "fuller" throughout the day, they also help to keep insulin levels more stable and under control. This also helps make your body much less prone to store excess fat.
- *Avoid eating meals in restaurants, or be more cautious when ordering food.* Restaurant food is typically high in calories, salt, and fat. Even if you try to order your meals without butter, oil, or salt, it's unlikely that they'll be served or prepared in the manner you request. You have to be very clear about how you would like your meal prepared, for example, "I'm allergic to butter and oil. If it's in my food, I'll barf. The last time it happened, I sued the chef, and the restaurant closed its doors." Never assume that the person preparing your food will abide by your wishes. Inspect your food before eating it, to be sure that it's made to your liking. In other words, be fussy, but in an agreeable way.
- *If there's no good reason for you to stay, don't hesitate to leave.* If you're not obligated to stay (that is, your mother or boss isn't there), gracefully make your exit (after using a preplanned excuse). Some of my friends use a beeper that they actually set off themselves.

"I'm sorry, I've got to go," they say, "my (kid, wife, or dog) is sick." When you're bored, or stressed, or anxious to leave, you tend to eat the wrong foods. Remember, if you don't have to stay, leaving may be your best bet.

10. NOT ADJUSTING TO SEASONAL OR HORMONAL VARIATIONS

For those of you who have SAD, are pregnant, or have PMS, it's important to pay attention to how these conditions affect how you eat. Refer to the sections in Chapter 5 (SAD and PMS), or speak to your doctor about your concerns if you're pregnant or postmenopausal. In addition, try using the points (for cravings and stress) revealed in this chapter.

Other Nutritional UFOs

- *Lack of emotional support.* You're ambushed by those who are envious of or threatened by your success (your efforts are often sabotaged by a spouse, family member, or friend). Others refuse to validate you or offer you any support.
- *Emotional hunger triggers and exacerbates physical hunger.* You may use food to console yourself, or to cover up difficult feelings.
- *Lack of healthy role models.*
- *Alcohol or drug abuse and/or a drug addiction.* See the Appendix for information regarding support groups and organizations.
- *Distorted body image.* Failing to identify or address an appearance obsession. Unfavorable comparisons to societal ideals.
- *Family history of issues involving your body image and food.* Examples are issues related to learned or conditioned patterns of eating, as well as self-image, feelings of guilt, and the role food has played in your family.
- *Lack of faith, either in yourself or in a higher power.* Failing to ask or to pray for support, believing that nothing will help.
- *Black-and-white thinking.* For example, "If I slip up once, I've failed."
- *Impatience.* Rapid-weight-loss diets lead to a slowed metabolic rate.

In addition, meal-replacement drinks are often high in carbs, which could cause your insulin levels to rise and your body to store more fat.

◆ *Desperate gullibility.* Seeking and trying the latest new diet or popular exercise fad.

◆ *Boredom, lack of direction.*

◆ *An abusive relationship history.* Often results in gaining weight to provide a "protective" shield.

◆ *Trusting unsupported claims by supplement manufacturers.* Buying into false promises.

◆ *Energy blocks.* Blocks involving feelings that relate to the way you eat.

◆ *Confusion that stems from exposure to varying theories, beliefs, and findings (with regard to diet programs and various experts' perspectives).*

PART III

Keys to Overcoming
Common Exercise UFOs

◆ ◆ ◆

Cardiovascular UFOs

Avoiding Common Obstacles to Peak Aerobic Fitness

In-san-i-ty n. Doing the same thing over and over, expecting a different result.

People watching is my business. Well, it's sort of my business. My living is made watching people work out and questioning how they behave. I wonder what people are thinking whenever I watch what they do in the gym. I see them on steppers, or stair machines, hunched over, with butts in the air, stressing their back, neck, and wrists in a way that's bound to be causing them pain. I see those who train the same way every day, without ever changing a thing, and can't understand why they're stuck in a rut or can't seem to lose any weight. I see people jumping on treadmills and bikes, without any warm-up at all, going like mad for a very short time and then just jumping right off. I see others joining their step classes late (and leaving without cooling down), who can't figure out why they never feel loose, or always end up getting hurt. I see lots of things, *some* that are good but most of them not good at all, and I ask myself, when people work out, what happens to their common sense? Why aren't they learning from all their mistakes? Why don't they ask for advice? Why do they do all these strange, silly things, when it's easy to see they don't help?

This chapter answers these questions in terms you can easily understand. It also exposes the reasons and ways that most people steer themselves wrong. By revealing the top ten UFOs that relate to aerobic fitness, it provides you with much of the insight you need to help you move past your blocks.

Top Ten Cardiovascular/Aerobic UFOs

1. A WARM-UP THAT'S INEFFICIENT, INCORRECT, OR POORLY PLANNED

The result is usually some type of injury, joint pain, weakness, or cramp, not to mention joint stiffness, decreased range of motion, and limited strength. It's too bad that so many people fail to warm up before they work out. It's as if it's not that important to them, or viewed as a tedious chore. Perhaps if you also avoid warming up, it's because you feel pressured for time. The irony, though, is that warming up right can actually *save* you time. First, because your muscles are much less apt to get achy or tight, you won't require as much rest between sets, meaning *less time* spent working out. You also avoid the frustration of having an injury hinder your gains. You save yourself all of the time you need to recover from tears and/or sprains.

I've also found people who do warm up either rush through the things that they do, or they perform useless movements (often in some type of hazardous way). Here are a few of the problems I see with the way that most people proceed.

◆ *Trying to stretch "cold" muscles*. Most people plop themselves down on a mat and stretch while their muscles are cold. Because of this, they often end up straining muscles and injuring joints. Always, before you begin to stretch, make sure that your muscles are warm. To insure that you do this correctly, consider the guidelines that follow:

◆ Perform a repetitive movement before you begin to stretch. Choose a non-weight-bearing exercise that won't overstress your joints. Also consider an exercise that involves your entire body. Some bikes and certain machines allow you to work with your upper arms, so when looking at warm-up options, you might want to keep this in mind. Other favorable options are elliptical cross-training steppers, walking with a pronounced arm swing, or rowing in an upright position. By performing a low-impact movement in which you use *all* of your large muscle groups, you increase the blood flow to your torso rather than just to your legs and hips.

◆ Exercise at an intensity that allows you to break a mild sweat. Your pulse should at least be twenty beats more than your typical resting rate.

◆ Regarding the duration, ten minutes should be the max. At least three minutes, and more often five, is the minimum most people need.

◆ *Inefficient stretching sequence.* Most people stretch their muscles in a random, perfunctory way. The way that we sequence our stretches, though, can be critical to our success. I suggest that you start your warm-up first by stretching your lower back. Because when performing most stretches, you do stress your lower back, it's best to target this area first, so it doesn't restrict other movements. Next, it's best to focus on parts of your body that give you a problem, like an area that you have injured before, or a muscle that tends to be tight. For example, if your hamstrings are tight, or prone to cramp up or tear, always stretch your hamstrings first before you stretch anything else. In addition, try *flexing* the muscle group that opposes the one that you'll stretch (for example, flex your hamstrings right before you start stretching your quads). When you contract the "antagonist" group before stretching targeted muscles, you "fool" the target group's stretch reflex and relax the muscle you're stretching. To ensure that your stretches are sequenced in the manner that serves you best, be sure to consider what follows when you plan your stretching routine:

In the past, Bill suffered some injuries to his triceps, quads, and chest. Because of this, his warm-up involves the following sequence of stretches:

— Warm-up (using an exercise bike that involves some use of the arms, keeping his torso upright and maintaining a comfortable pace).

— Lower back stretches (that don't place much stress on his biceps, his quads, or his chest).

— A hamstring contraction (held 5–10 seconds), and then, a quadriceps stretch.

— A lat and/or shoulder contraction (held 5–10 seconds), and then, a chest stretch.

— A biceps contraction (held 5–10 seconds), and then, a triceps stretch.

Then, the following muscle groups (stretching the larger of these groups first):

Glutes/buttocks
Shoulders (deltoids)
Neck
Calves

Antagonist Muscle Group Pairings
◆ quadriceps and hamstrings
◆ erector spinae (lower back) and abdominals
◆ triceps and biceps
◆ calves and anterior tibialis (shin)
◆ deltoids (shoulders), pectoralis major (chest), and/or latissimus dorsi (upper back)

◆ *Performing stretches improperly, in a hurried, cursory fashion.* Most people rush through their stretching routine as if it's a tedious task. They don't hold their stretches long enough to benefit much from their effort. They also don't take enough time to assume an effective stretching position. And most tend to bounce or to "pulse," as opposed to properly holding each stretch. The guidelines that I most often suggest, very briefly, are as follows.

◆ Never bounce or "pulse" when you stretch (avoid all "ballistic" movement).
◆ Always perform stretches "statically," which means you must hold every stretch.

- Perform all your stretches slowly; move gradually into position.
- Hold each stretch thirty seconds (or longer if muscles are tight).
- Contract the *antagonist* muscle group first, before stretching targeted groups. For example, if stretching your triceps, contract your biceps first. This will "switch off" your stretch reflex, relaxing the muscle you're stretching.
- Repeat any stretches that challenge you, or involve muscle groups that are tight.
- Avoid any forward flexion when you stretch in a standing position (if you bend forward when you're standing, your lower back is at risk).

◆ *Failing to hold each stretch for a long enough time to derive any gain.* A study that was reported in a physical therapy journal revealed that about thirty seconds is the best time to hold a stretch. Fifty-seven participants who took part in a six-week study found that holding a stretch for less time produced less effective results. They also discovered that when a stretch was held for sixty seconds, it helped no more than holding a stretch for half that amount of time. By holding your stretches for more (or less) time, you can see for yourself what works best. You may find that some of your muscle groups need a longer, more thorough stretch.

◆ *Muscles stretched during the warm-up will get tight again if they're not used.* One of the problems with stretching your muscles *only* before you work out is that most are apt to get tight again well before you stress them with weights. If you train your calves with weights, for example, *well after* you do your calf stretches, you're likely to find that your calf muscles are no longer warm or loose. If you don't work your calves right after you stretch, your calf stretches won't do much good. That's why I have my clients perform, for example, a quadriceps stretch, just prior to when they start training their quads, and then, once again, when they're done. As long as they're held thirty seconds or more, for some people, one stretch will do. I rarely see anyone doing this, though, which is strange, since it makes perfect sense. A muscle that's stretched will be stronger than one that is tight, or that isn't warmed-up.

◆ *Inappropriate stretches:*

- ◆ *Yoga plough:* compression of discs and vertebrae, strain on the lower back.
- ◆ *Hurdler's stretch:* increased potential for knee strain with the leg in the hurdler's position.
- ◆ *Butterfly (groin) stretch:* bouncy, "ballistic" movement increases the strain on the knees and the groin.
- ◆ *Toe touches or forward flexion when in a standing position:* potentially hazardous stress on the muscles and discs of the lower back.
- ◆ *Lower back hyperextension:* disc compression.
- ◆ *Standing quadriceps stretch:* a tendency to "yank" the targeted leg into stretching position increases the chance of a muscle tear and/or strain to the back or the knees.

2. MISUNDERSTANDING HOW DIFFERENT APPROACHES AFFECT METABOLIC EFFICIENCY

Conventional wisdom tells us that the best way to burn more fat is to do cardiovascular exercise at a slower and less intense pace. The theory is that because when we exercise hard we use glucose for fuel, if we exercise at a more moderate pace, we'll draw from our fat stores instead. If you've always believed this to be the case, you can pat yourself on the back. It's true that we tend to burn slightly more fat when we train at a less-intense pace. Nevertheless, this fact is distorted in terms of its truth and importance. Actually, even though *while you work out* a slower pace burns more fat, when you exercise more intensely you burn more fat *once you stop*. Because you're increasing your fat-burning rate, and it also stays higher for longer, working out more intensely yields more fat-burning *after the fact*. The difference, then, is negligible and the net result is the same. Whether your workout is short and intense or longer and more slowly paced, you end up burning just as much fat, but simply at different times.

A researcher from Georgia State, physiologist Jeffrey Rupp, conducted a study comparing fat loss via different approaches to training. He found that when two groups of women walked on a treadmill for almost three months, both the high- and low-effort groups burned an equal amount of fat. Both groups trained four times a week, until they burned 300 calories. While the fast walkers usually burned this amount in thirty minutes or less, the slow walkers needed in general about forty to fifty-five. Both groups reduced their fat 3 percent and ended up just as fit.

The verdict? Do whatever feels best to you, or vary the way you train. Either way, stop fretting so much about finding new ways to burn fat. Doing what's best for your body should be your first and foremost concern.

3. IMPROPER USE OF EQUIPMENT

Equipment adjustments are either not made or made in an improper fashion. Common examples:

- Adjusting the seat on an exercise bike so it's either too high or too low. When seated, with feet on the pedals and with your torso positioned upright, your extended leg should be slightly bent (you should never straighten your knees).
- Adjusting the grade on the treadmill to a position that stresses the back. When the grade is higher than thirty degrees it can strain your lower back (those who suffer with lower back pain *should not* assume inclined positions).

Most people train with poor technique, or train in awkward positions. Common examples:

- Leaning forward on step machines, with the back excessively arched.
- Failing to stay in an upright position when stepping or using a bike. This places stress on your hands and wrists, causing numbness, weakness, and pain.
- Working out on a step machine with a rapid, restricted motion (moving with short, hurried, choppy steps instead of throughout a full range).
- Failing to stay in an upright position when using a rowing machine. Leaning too far forward places stress on the lower back.

4. FAILURE TO VARY THE TRAINING MODE

Are you a creature of habit? Do you stick with the things that you like? If this is the case, and you're not making gains, it's time to find more things you like. It's critical that when you exercise, you vary the things you do. Not only because you're apt to get bored, but also because you'll get "stale." This happens because your body adapts to familiar patterns of stress. If you don't change the way you exercise, you may never observe further gains.

It's no more complex than that. Vary your mode of training at least every two to three weeks. That way, you won't get complacent doing the same old familiar thing. You'll also ensure that your efforts are always resulting in optimum gains.

Sample Weekly Routine

Monday: Exercise bike, maintaining your target heart rate (THR) for twenty-five minutes.

Wednesday: Step machine, maintaining your THR for thirty minutes.

Friday: Step aerobics, maintaining your THR for forty minutes.

Continue this cycle for two to three weeks, then consider the following options: Vary your modes of training (try rowing, jogging, or swimming); keep one or two of the same training modes but do them on different days; or add another session to your weekly aerobic routine.

It's also important to vary the time and intensity of your routines. On certain days you may choose to work hard for a shorter amount of time. On other days you may want to increase your duration and lessen your pace. The key is to "trick" your body to make sure that it "stays on its toes." You don't want it getting too comfortable with whatever it is you do. If you vary both the intensity and the duration of your routines (in addition to changing their frequency and the manner in which you train), you are doing everything possible to ensure that your progress persists.

5. AN OBSESSION WITH BURNING CALORIES

The subject of calorie burning rarely fails to get our attention. These days, it's highly unlikely that you can read any magazine without seeing some information regarding what training modes burn the most fat. There's often a list of various modes of cardiovascular training, with every exercise rated in terms of its calorie-burning potential (CBP). Because for so many folks the CBP is the foremost concern, most people favor the exercise modes with the highest CBPs. It's actually this type of mind-set that is often a UFO. It makes people do things they shouldn't do, things that aren't right for their body. For example, if some expert claims that we burn more calories climbing stairs, overweight folks with bad backs and bad knees will be anxious to start climbing stairs. It's time that we found a way to curb our calorie-burning fixation. Instead, we must do what *feels* best instead of what burns the most fat. Better to walk—and enjoy it—and burn just a little less fat than to follow the latest new fat-burning trend and to quit when you find it's too hard.

Rating exercise modes this way is misleading anyway. It assumes that we all tend to move and perform in exactly the same type of way. It also assumes that we're all predisposed to burn fat at a similar rate and doesn't account for the fact that our levels of fitness and builds aren't the same. The amount of calories burned when you train depends on many factors, including your ratio of muscle to fat and what groups of muscles you use. The larger the groups that you use the most, the more fat you're likely to burn.

6. OVERTRAINING

This is a problem that's actually much more common than people think. Many folks think that by failing to exercise most every day of the week, they'll either be forced to accept being fat or be forced to eat like a bird. This is what's called being paranoid, if this fact isn't already clear. In general, you'll be overtrained if you train *more than five times a week*. You'll also be overtraining if you exceed your target heart rate, or if you stay in your target zone for forty-five minutes or more. If you exercise too much longer than this, it may hurt you more than it helps. You'll be prone to overuse injuries and have less motivation to train. Moreover, there's little to gain from performing additional weekly sessions. Even if you trained every day, and never got injured or bored, your efforts would probably fail to reap any kind of worthwhile reward. Overtraining aerobically can cause shin splints and tendonitis, as well as sciatica, knee strain, heel spurs, back strain, and exercise slumps. The irony is that if you're a person who frequently overtrains, you may end up *undertrained*, because you'll be more predisposed to get hurt. Your training won't be consistent enough to allow for continued progress.

Cardiovascular Training Intensity
For optimum benefit, 70–85 percent of your maximum heart rate (220–your age).
70 percent if you're sedentary or in poor to fair condition
75 percent if you're fit but in only average shape
80 percent if you're fairly fit (in better than average shape)
85 percent if you're very fit or training for competition

Simple Equation for Determining Your Target (Aerobic) Heart Rate
THR = 220–Your Age × .7 to .85 (depending on your fitness level)

7. UNDERTRAINING

Here's the general rule of thumb with regard to aerobic exercise: Undertraining is exercising *fewer than three times a week*, or not maintaining your THR for at least twenty minutes per session. When your body is undertrained, it's also underchallenged. To improve your aerobic fitness to a point that's considered ideal, your heart rate must be consistently at or above your THR (more than 70 percent of 220–your age). If your heart rate when training is lower than this, you won't make significant gains. You may feel a little bit better and be somewhat more physically fit, but because you improve so slowly, you're apt to get fed up and quit. It's better to work in the optimum range for improving your level of fitness. The higher your level of fitness, the higher your heart rate should be.

8. INCONSISTENT INTENSITY

For years, we've listened to experts say that the key to getting in shape is maintaining the target heart rate for at least twenty minutes per session. Now some say that interval training may help just as much. Soon we'll hear that some other approach has been found to be more effective, and then, once we've all bought into it, we'll be urged to try something else. How can we know for sure, then, that we're doing what serves us best? Should we stick to the old fitness formulas, or should we try some new-fashioned approach?

Throughout this book, my advice has reflected what *I* have found to be true, not just what the research reveals, or what experts insist is the case. In keeping with this, what I suggest with regard to aerobic training is that, as a rule, you do your best to maintain your THR. I've found as I've worked with clients over the course of fifteen years, that those who maintain their THR progress at the fastest rates. For most, a consistent THR is the key to aerobic success. But it seems as if people don't realize, or fail to acknowledge, that this is true. Most exercise so frenetically that their heart rate is rarely maintained. As a result, they don't challenge their body enough to achieve their goals. They would benefit more if they exercised at a more consistent pace. It would help them to burn more calories as well as to be more fit.

Assessing Your Training Intensity

Check your training heart rate. Heart rate checks are invaluable when you're first beginning to train. It helps you to know, without question, if you're working as hard as you should. In addition, heart rate checks can help if you're trying a new mode of training, by providing you with an objective view of the way your body responds. The problem, though, is that most people have a hard time feeling their pulse, or, when they slow down to take it, their pulse rate abruptly declines. This is why pulse rate monitors are such valuable fitness tools. Those that are most effective attach with a strap just below your chest and tend to be fairly accurate compared to other pulse-taking methods. *Polar* pulse rate monitors are considered among the best, but it's wise to ask those who have used them before about which types they recommend. (For purchasing information, refer to the Appendix.)

Perceived levels of exertion. To perceive your exertion correctly, you should already be in good shape. Beginners, who aren't as attuned to the way that a workout makes them feel, are less apt to have an accurate sense of their effort when they start to train. In part, this explains why so many folks initially work too hard. If you work out consistently and are accustomed to how it feels, perceiving your level of effort is an option that makes good sense.

Modified Perceived Exertion Rating Scale

Rate yourself on the following scale to determine how hard you should train. If you're just starting out, aim for a 3; if active, aim for a 4.

1: A mild degree of effort, with little appreciable stress. You can speak without having to catch your breath, and your muscles are under no strain.

2: Your exercise level is comfortable; your body feels minimally challenged. Your respiration has slightly increased, and it's not difficult to speak.

3: You're breathing noticeably faster, and more aware of how you feel. You can speak, but it's not quite as easy to do, and you're starting to break a sweat. Your muscles feel somewhat challenged, but you know you could handle more. You're only a little bit winded. You're maintaining a moderate pace.

4: You're moving at a spirited pace but still not going all-out. Your body is being challenged, but you still can maintain your effort. You no longer can speak comfortably, and you're starting to break a good sweat. Your respiration has increased quite a bit, and your muscles are feeling some stress. You're working as hard as you possibly can without feeling as if it's *too* hard.

5: You can feel your heart pounding vigorously, and you're starting to gasp for air. You can't speak more than a few quick words, and your muscles are starting to ache. You couldn't push any harder than this for more than a very short time.

9. POOR TIMING

I'm often surprised when people reveal what they do before they work out. "I just finished lunch" or "I went without lunch" are comments that I often hear. I also hear statements like, "Boy, am I pooped, I haven't had any sleep," or "Gee, I always feel tired whenever I put in a twelve-hour day." Granted, these things do happen. But it's when they happen consistently that it's important to find out why. Here's the problem, in general, with each of these typical UFOs:

Whenever you've just completed a meal, your body shunts blood to your gut. If you exercise on a full stomach without giving food time to digest, you're making your muscles compete with your stomach in order to get enough blood. This impedes your digestion, as well as the way you train.

If you go a long time without eating, your blood sugar level declines. This can make you feel weak, fatigued, and light-headed when you're working out.

If you exercise with little sleep, or train when your rhythm is off, you'll be less energetic and much less enthusiastic about working out.

If you exercise at the end of the day, when your body and mind are fatigued, your energy level is apt to be low and you won't be inspired to train. If it's okay with you and your body, try training first thing when you wake. If you're able to train as soon as you rise, without feeling worse for the wear, you'll tap your fat stores for energy rather than burning up glucose for fuel.

Some folks always perform their aerobic routines before they lift weights. Their rationale is that it's best to perform cardiovascular exercise first, as it loosens up joints and ensures that their muscles aren't stressed when they're still cold or tight. Only in very rare instances, though, do I feel that this serves people best. Here's my take on the matter, based on what I routinely observe. Because when you train with weights, it's so important to use proper form, it makes more sense to weight-train first, when your energy is at its peak. If your energy is depleted, you're less apt to use good technique. Your movements tend to be less controlled, and your joints are more apt to be weak. Moreover, you'll find it hard to ensure that your muscles are fully fatigued. Those who reject this point of view and who work out aerobically first usually don't understand, or accept, the value of training to failure. Because they perform an arbitrary or comfortable number of reps, it doesn't matter so much that before they begin they're already fatigued. They always perform the same number of reps, if their muscles are tired or not.

When you perform an aerobic routine after you work out with weights, as long as your legs aren't extremely fatigued, you shouldn't be hindered at all. You shouldn't have trouble maintaining your pace, unless you work out very hard. I recommend that when possible you train different ways, different days—for example, a weight workout three times a week and aerobics on alternate days. Or split up your workouts to allow for some rest in between. When forced to do them together, though, in general do weight training first, unless when training with weights your intensity level is usually low.

10. IGNORING YOUR LIMITATIONS OR NOT TRAINING "RIGHT FOR YOUR TYPE"

When it comes to choosing an exercise mode that is likely to serve them best, too many people fail to consider their physical limitations. Even if they have an injury that precludes certain types of movement, many folks favor what's "trendy" over what actually makes the most sense. It's important to choose the exercise modes that are best for your body and mind. For example, if you have knee problems, or problems involving your feet, jogging or slide aerobics probably aren't your safest bet. Something like water aerobics is a far more practical choice. In addition, besides taking into account what is best for your type of body, you should think about how different exercise modes are accustomed to making you feel. To determine what factors you should keep in mind when choosing a method of training, refer to Chapter 7 (fitness and body type classifications).

Weight-Training UFOs

Ensuring a Flawless Workout

We need exercise in order to die young as old as possible.

—Heinz W. Lenz

I have this recurring nightmare. First I'm chained to a step machine and then I'm bound and gagged. Then I'm forced to watch people hurt themselves while they're working out. But the worst part is that I live this dream whenever I go to the gym. You see, I tend to get very upset when I see the things most people do. Actually, it's the sounds they make that bother me most of all. Over and over again, wherever I go, it's always the same: plates slamming, machines clanging, weights crashing to the floor—an uninterrupted cacophony of clamorous, nerve-rattling noise. If you've ever listened to somebody scratching a metal pan with a fork, you probably can relate to the way this usually makes me feel.

Please don't get me wrong. I'm happy to see people trying in the best way they know how, but I think I now know how my shop teacher felt when he saw me pound nails with a wrench. When the wrong tools are used the wrong way for the job, it can look and sound pretty ugly. And it also gets done very poorly.

Granted, this job isn't easy. Present-day theories on how to lift weights are diverse, to say the least. With so many folks saying so many things, it's hard to know what to trust, especially when the advice they give is put in technical terms. We often assume that the bigger the words, the more factual they must be. But we must bear in mind that what *sounds* best may not always be what *is* best. More technical and/ or more eloquent does not always mean more valid.

In this chapter, you identify your weight training UFOs. You are introduced to the FOCUS Technique, a unique new way of training, and are shown how to use this simple technique to overcome common blocks. In addition, you learn new ways to achieve your muscular fitness potential, as well as how long, how hard, and how much you must train to accomplish your goals.

◆ **EXERCISE** ◆

Assessing Your Training Technique: Are You Doing What Serves You Best?

—— Are you certain that your training technique is efficient, safe, and effective? Do you have objective evidence to support your point of view?

—— Have you taken the time to consult with those who have used different methods of training?

—— Have you ever tracked your progress using various types of techniques?

—— Have you ever compared, in an unbiased way, dissimilar methods of training?

Scoring

If you've answered these questions honestly, and at least one answer is no, there's a pretty good chance you've experienced some type of weight-training UFO.

◆ ◆ ◆

How can you keep from falling prey to poor or misleading advice? In short, you must be objective. Always be open to different ideas and varying points of view, but be sure to assess them thoroughly before you decide on a major change. Remember to always ask questions about whatever you don't understand. By asking appropriate questions, you'll avoid being led astray. You'll be able to see more clearly the type of approach that will serve you best.

Altering Egos

Imagine how you might feel if your ego suddenly ceased to exist. Life would be very different, in quite a few ways, don't you think? Just imagine, no keeping up with the Joneses, no one you have to impress, even the time that you spend at the gym would involve less competitive stress. Imagine yourself being less concerned about how you compared to others, acknowledging your limitations and being careful not to exceed them, learning to find success in ways that you never believed you could! If you're like most people, perhaps you agree that it would be a welcome change.

When people are led by their ego, they do things that hinder their gains. For example, quite often when people work out, they use much more weight than they should. They don't understand that they do so at a considerable expense. They increase their risk of injury and restrict their rate of success.

I learned this the hard way. There was a time when I almost always trained with very heavy weights, performing each movement as rapidly and as explosively as I could. I thought that the more I "worked up a sweat," the more I stood to gain. I didn't have any idea that there was a better, and safer, approach.

All along I was confident that what I was doing was right, partly because I did observe a certain amount of improvement. But it wasn't as much as I'd hoped for, and the price I paid was high. I was always tired, often injured, and rarely inspired to work out. Still, although I was conscious of this, I refused to consider a change. I worried that if I did, I'd promptly lose what little I'd gained. I was also much too proud to admit that what I was doing was wrong. My ego was much too fragile.

As time passed, and little changed, I was forced to admit the truth: I was moving much too quickly and using excessive amounts of weight. The result was very discouraging but not at all uncommon. I experienced quite a bit of *pain* but achieved very little *gain*.

The FOCUS Technique: The Ultimate Weight-Training Formula

I realized that to achieve success, I would have to slow myself down. *A lot*. In fact, if you read the instructions on the machines at your health club or gym, you'll see that they say to move *slowly*, in a strict and focused fashion. Truth be told, the word "slowly" is misunderstood by most folks who lift weights. Actually, slowly means very slow, much slower than most people think. It may even mean much slower than you've heard most instructors advise.

If you're relating to any of this (and I'm guessing you probably are), it will benefit you to rethink your approach with regard to the following rule: To ensure that your efforts are always safe, efficient, sound, and effective, all of your movements must be performed in a slow and deliberate manner. They must be Fluid, Optimally Controlled, and, especially, Ultra-Slow. The value of this approach, referred to henceforth as the FOCUS Technique, cannot be overstated with regard to achieving success. It is critical to ensuring both a safe and effective result.

Perfecting a FOCUS movement may require a little practice. It isn't always as easy or as simple as it seems. If, after reading further, you decide to employ this technique, be warned that it may feel awkward at first, quite different from what you do now. But rest assured that with patience your efforts are sure to pay off.

Timing the Lift

In general, when you're lifting a weight, experts recommend this: That you raise the weight to a count of two and lower to a count of four. They advise that a movement's lowering phase should be *half the speed* of the lift. Although it makes sense to lower a weight at a less rapid rate of speed, I don't believe that it's wise to adhere to the "2-4" recommendation, mostly because different movements have very different ranges of motion. To complete each rep of each exercise in exactly six seconds time (two seconds up, four seconds down), you'd actually have to move *faster* to execute lifts with a *wider* range.

You would also have to move *slower* in order to execute those that were *shorter*. Given these facts, to use the same count on each exercise makes little sense.

To understand the difference, it may help to consider this. Imagine performing an exercise with a very limited range (e.g., the shoulder shrug) compared to performing a movement with a considerably wider range (the pullover). If you performed both movements in the same exact span of time (six seconds), you'd have to perform the pullover *fast* and the shoulder shrug *very slowly*. Instead, both movements should be performed at the same slow rate of speed.

You may also have heard that a weight should be lowered more slowly than it is raised. This guideline is given primarily: (1) to lessen the use of momentum (by lifting, not "swinging," a weight); (2) to encourage a more controlled movement; and (3) to stress muscles more intensely during the lowering phase of a rep. But although most people know that they should move "slower whenever they lower," even the most conscientious folks will rarely move slowly enough. In fact, they should lower *and* lift a weight much slower than they ever do.

To correctly perform the FOCUS Technique, consider the following rule: While the lifting phase of most movements should be *four to six* seconds long, the duration of the lowering phase should be roughly *six to eight*. This depends on the exercise as well as the range of motion.

Moving this slowly might seem extreme compared to what you've seen. You may even think, "if it works so well, then why doesn't everyone do it?" The primary reason, in my view, is that few realize the advantage. Few even know that training this way is an option they should consider! Some claim they get the concept but don't want to risk looking strange. They're afraid to be unconventional, regardless of what they might gain.

Although others may try to dissuade you, I urge you to give this a try. If you're willing to give it a fair enough chance, your progress will speak for itself.

How You Know You're Moving Too Fast

- You mostly feel stress on your joints or on inappropriate parts of your body.
- You're stressing the target muscle group (prime mover), but only at certain points.
- You're consistently moving or tensing inappropriate parts of your body (for example, shrugging your shoulders or arching your back while performing a curl).
- You're consistently holding your breath.
- You can't stabilize your position or have problems maintaining your balance.
- You fail to achieve isolation of the muscle you want to target.
- You're moving your body consistently in a jerky, explosive fashion.

How You Know You're Moving Too Slowly

- You're not improving your technique at all by moving any more slowly.
- You're concerned more about moving "perfectly" than with performing a maximum effort.
- You're not exercising consistently in a fluid, steady manner.
- You tend to stop or to take short rests between and during repetitions.

To give you a sense of how to perform an efficient FOCUS movement, imagine performing a plié (slow knee bend often performed as a warm-up) or the motions involved in tai chi. A FOCUS movement, correctly performed, is essentially much the same. Every motion is graceful, focused, slow, and well controlled. Every movement is safe, precise, and optimally effective.

Unquestionably, moving slowly is just good common sense. Unfortunately, not everyone is so easy to convince. I was once approached by a man who worked out regularly at my gym. He said he'd been training for more than six years but had failed to reach most of his goals. After speaking to him for a very short time, it was clear that he needed help.

I informed him about the benefits of employing the FOCUS Technique. Confident that he'd see for himself, I convinced him to give it a try. He was clearly very surprised. "I can't believe it," he said to me. "My muscles feel so much more pumped! I can really feel the difference! What you said is really true!"

I went on to tell him more about the importance of moving slowly. "Maybe you're right," he promptly replied, "but I couldn't train that way. I could never move that slowly. I'm just not patient enough."

"Hmmm," I thought, as I paused to consider his honest but puzzling response. "He says that he isn't patient enough to train in a more controlled way, *but* he's patient enough to train the same way *for six years* without making gains!"

Too often, we do what is common instead of what makes the most sense. This is because it's so hard for us to risk doing things that are new. By clinging to what is familiar, though, we take a much greater risk. We risk facing ongoing UFOs and falling far short of our goals.

Less Is More

To perform an exercise slowly, you have to use less weight. How much less? To start, try using 60 percent of the amount you normally use. Remember, it's not *how much* you use, it's *how you use it* that counts. In fact, when employing the FOCUS Technique, using *less* weight helps you *more*. Although you might worry that if you do you'll feel like you're losing ground, by moving more slowly and strictly, you're really *advancing* the way you train. Once you've witnessed the difference, you're apt to abandon your doubts.

Consider Sue's experience. Sue was a fitness devotee who'd been training hard for years. But despite her diligent efforts, she had failed to accomplish her goals. She was also hampered by injuries and, more often than not, was in pain. It seemed that no matter what she did, very little seemed to change.

"I've been trying as hard as I can," Sue said, "but not much has happened at all. I've tried everything I can think of, but my body refuses to budge. It's been an unending struggle for me, more trouble by far than it's worth. Sometimes I feel like just giving up, like simply accepting the truth—that despite all my time and effort, working out isn't working out!"

While watching Sue as she huffed and puffed through a typical daily routine, it was easy to see that her careless technique was the crux of what held her back. Much as I had suspected, she was training with too much weight. She was also moving much too fast and not stabilizing her joints. I suggested a slower and stricter approach (the FOCUS Technique), which she promptly agreed to try.

After training this way for only three months, Sue's body had fully transformed. Her muscles were taut and shapely and significantly more defined. In addition, her posture was much improved, and she rarely had *any* discomfort. Inspired by her improvement, she decided to try a new diet. She succeeded in lowering her body fat from 30 to 16 percent.

"It's incredible," Sue said, shaking her head, still finding it hard to believe. "Lifting a weight very slowly is more important than most people think! When I do, I feel that my body is able to be more in sync with my mind. The best part, though, is because what I'm doing is clearly so much more efficient, I no longer have to do so many sets, and I don't have to train for so long. I even spend less time in the gym and feel better when I leave. Now I can't even imagine myself working out any other way. You just have to learn to FOCUS—it's amazing how well it works!"

As a personal trainer, I like to build a rapport with those I instruct. While getting to know a new client, I asked why she wanted my help. I tried on my bathing suit, she explained. It's a thong—but it's not supposed to be.

—MONICA PRICE

Intensity and Movement Speed

Of course, working out at a slow rate of speed is a far cry from the norm. In fact, I'm often questioned by those who don't understand its value. "Why do you move so slowly," they ask, "when fast movements are more intense?" It's really too bad they see it this way. They couldn't be more off the mark. I guess that because I'm not grunting a lot or heaving some ponderous weight, it doesn't appear that I'm working out hard or expending a whole lot of effort. But working out "hard" means working out "right," in ways that are safe and efficient. The *only* way to train properly is to move slowly when lifting a weight.

The reality is that when most people train, they technically aren't "lifting" weights. Instead, they're actually "throwing" them. Weight "throwers" move explosively. They use the heaviest weight they can, in *any way* they can. Because they use momentum when performing all of their movements, they fail to stress their muscles throughout a maximum range of motion.

Weight "lifters" know that to exercise hard they must also exercise right. They know that when *lifting* ten pounds in a slow and fluid fashion, they are actually training harder than when *throwing* fifty pounds fast. They know that to raise their intensity they must stress only target muscles, not mostly tendons and ligaments or vulnerable parts of their body.

Flexibility and Movement Speed

The FOCUS Technique has another plus: There's much less chance you'll get hurt. When lifting weights conventionally (in a vigorous, rapid fashion), joints are more likely to weaken, and muscles are more apt to tear. This happens much like a rubber band frays when it's pulled and released very fast (pull and release it slowly, though, and you'll see that it *doesn't* fray). When a fiber frays, or repeatedly tears, the result can be quite severe: Scar tissue builds, adhesions form, and muscles become very tight. In fact, the reason why muscle-bound folks are inflexible, as a rule, is not that they are constrained by their muscles or hampered some way by their size. They are usually hindered by scar tissue that's resulted from fast, jerky lifts.

> *Now almost all of my movements are slower and more precise. By attempting to lift very heavy weights in a rapid, explosive fashion, you fail to isolate muscles enough to achieve significant gains. Explosive lifts cause muscle tears and overstressed, weakened joints. I was beginning to experience the consequences.*
>
> —DORIAN YATES, PROFESSIONAL BODYBUILDER AND
> MR. OLYMPIA WINNER

Cheating

Why do people so often train in a rapid, uncontrolled fashion? Mostly because when doing so, they're able to use more weight. But it's clear that this builds the ego quite a bit more than it does the body. While it's true that lifting a heavy weight can provide an emotional boost, this doesn't mean we can disregard its potential for causing us harm.

Second, most lack the patience to focus on using a slower technique. Even when they agree that moving slowly makes more sense, they worry that it'll take more time, or simply be too hard to do. What they fail to see, though, is that if they moved more slowly, they could actually perform far fewer sets and achieve far better results. As a result, it's probable that they'd finish their workout *faster* (performing one set slowly takes less time than two done fast).

Some people feel, on occasion, that it serves them to use faulty form (cheating). They say that it helps to force a weight past the hardest parts of a movement, so that different parts of a movement range can be more thoroughly stressed. I'm not convinced that this "benefit" really makes cheating worth the risk. No matter how you look at it, the cons outweigh the pros. When cheating, you change your technique in a way that increases your injury risk (for example, by shrugging your shoulders or arching your back when performing a curl). Doing so places much of the stress on vulnerable parts of your body.

Top Ten "More Appropriate" Names for Common Error-Prone Movements

1. Arching Chest Bounce (bench press)
2. Jerky Dumbbell Fling (lateral raise)
3. Shrugging Barbell Throw (standing biceps curl)
4. Buttocks Elevation (push-up)
5. Seated High-Speed Cable Yank (seated row or pulldown)
6. Jerk-up (pull-up or sit-up)
7. Plate Banging, Rump-Raised Leg Whip (prone hamstring curl)
8. Rapid Bent-Legged Calf Jiggle (calf raise)

9. Very Slight Supine Head Raise (abdominal crunch)
10. Really Fast Seated Leg Swing (leg extension)

Fast Versus Slow Movements

Many believe that working out fast is the optimum way to build strength. They also believe that by doing so they'll build more muscle mass. They base their beliefs, in part, on the fact that muscles have two types of fibers. (In fact, there are four variations of types, each with a different function. But here, just to keep things simple, I refer to the two basic types.) Fast-twitch, or white muscle, fibers are mostly employed for feats of strength. They're used when performing activities that are primarily anaerobic, such as those that require explosive, quick bursts of strength, like a jump or a sprint. Slow-twitch, or red muscle, fibers are primarily used for endurance. They're used when performing activities that are considered to be aerobic, such as long-distance running and swimming, cycling, rowing, or long "power" walks.

Many assume that *fast* fibers are triggered mostly by *faster* movements. Because we use more fast fibers to perform movements requiring strength, they believe that weight training should be performed at a rapid rate of speed.

At first glance, this seems to make sense. Fast movements, one might imagine, would primarily stress fast fibers. Conversely, it might seem logical that slow movements should stress slower fibers. But the role of different fiber types is not quite this simplistic. It's the *intensity*, not the movement speed, that determines which fibers are used. Put simply, the harder that muscles must work, the more you'll employ fast fibers. Slow movements, performed with heavy weights, affect fiber types that are *fast*.

Regardless of whether moving fast is in any way effective, the risk you take when doing so is too serious to ignore. Research shows that moving fast increases your risk of injury by increasing the compressive and sheer force affecting muscles, tendons, and joints. In addition, moving a heavy weight fast increases abdominal pressure, which results in a higher blood pressure than is considered safe when you train.

Though the value of training at slower speeds is supported by numerous studies, there was one of particular interest conducted in the winter of 1995. The study, revealed in the winter edition of *Nautilus* magazine, was directed by Dr. Wayne Wescott, who consults for the YMCA. Wescott enlisted six women, ages eighteen to thirty-six, who were tested to see how their gains in strength were related to movement speed. While performing the leg extension (over a nine-week span of time), they trained one leg at a slow speed (60 degrees per second) and the other comparably fast (240 degrees per second). To understand the difference, it will help to consider this: To extend your leg at a speed of 240 degrees per second, it would take less than half a second for you to complete the lifting phase. Conversely, you would need four times as long (at 60 degrees per second).

The results of the test clearly favored performing a weight-training movement slowly. While each subject's fast-trained leg showed virtually no improvement at all, the strength of the slow-trained leg increased an average of 9 percent. Bear in mind also that this was when tested at *both* slow and rapid speeds.

Although there have been many studies performed to evaluate movement speed, there is still very little agreement about what actually works the best. Research is often distorted, in fact, to support one's personal bias. Given that this is the case, I strongly suggest that you heed this advice: Regardless of what you read or hear, do what feels right for *you*. Always use your common sense, but above all, trust your instincts. If something doesn't *feel* right, the odds are it's probably not.

If fifty million people say a foolish thing, it is still a foolish thing.
—ANATOLE FRANCE

Paced Resistance Exercises

Traditionally, exercise classes include a segment of "spot toning" movements. You may also have heard these movements referred to as "floor work" or "isolations." They're often performed by instructors during the last phase of a class, at a pace that's determined, in large part, by the selection of music that's used. While it may be true that music can make an exercise class more fun, it cannot be considered appropriate when one weighs the pros and cons. More often than not, in an exercise class, it involves considerable risk.

A resistance movement shouldn't be "paced" by a fixed or programmed rhythm. Here's why. When muscles go *anaerobic*, they quickly become fatigued. If at this point you start *forcing* yourself to maintain a consistent speed, the muscles that you begin to use most are those you should use least. In effect, you fail to isolate the muscles you're hoping to target. This is what happens in classes. Typically, people strain themselves in an effort to follow the beat. But as they continue to do this (and their muscles become more fatigued), they usually start to move in a way that defeats what they're trying to do (for example, arching their back or jerking and flailing their arms and legs). This is very likely to lead to some type of serious harm.

Movements performed *aerobically* require less muscular effort. As a result, they can be sustained without reaching muscular failure. Performing these movements to music, besides being safer, makes better sense.

Performing High Numbers of Reps to Promote and Target the Loss of Fat

Now for a little myth debunking. Did you know that using a very light weight and performing numerous reps will not do very much to improve your muscular definition? If you're able to do more than fifteen reps before reaching muscular failure, you're not working out intensely enough to achieve any meaningful gains. Despite what you may have heard and read (or been told by a well-meaning trainer), you won't see much improvement in either the tone or the shape of your muscles. Nor will a high-repetition approach do much to increase your strength. For all but a few rare exceptions, the intensity is too low.

In addition, many subscribe to the view that the best way to spot reduce is to target "problem areas" such as the abdomen, buttocks, and thighs. Many believe that to do so they must perform "isolation" movements, such as hip adductions/abductions, ab crunches, leg lifts, side bends, or twists. If you share this common perspective, there is something you should know: These movements target muscle groups, not deposits of fat. There's no way to burn or break down fat in just one part of the body. That's not the way exercise works.

Very seldom are problem spots the result of poorly toned muscles. For example, your abs are rarely less toned than other parts of your body. Problem areas simply are those that happen to be fat-prone. If you overtrain the muscle groups that underlie these areas, you may very well find to your dismay that these areas increase in size! So if you intend to reduce your waist, and you do lots of side bends and twists, while you might build a little muscle, you'll lose no fat at all. The result? More girth to your waist.

If you have succeeded in losing fat from a certain part of your body, it's not because you've done countless reps of an "adipose-burning" movement. Unfortunately, despite what you've heard, no such thing exists. The key to your success was increasing your ratio of muscle to fat.

Instead of performing so many sets (and reps) of a certain movement, take more steps to improve how you eat and to boost your aerobic fitness. Focus more on reducing fat, not overtraining your muscles.

Safety First

In order for any exercise to be truly safe and effective, you must always pay strict attention to your movement range and speed. If you move too fast or too far for too long, you're apt to experience pain. And if a movement is painful for you, or is awkward for you to perform, it's a pretty good bet that at some point you're going to end up getting hurt.

It's important that when you exercise your movements are always fluid. There should be a natural rhythm and flow that resonates with your body. When an exercise is performed properly (when using the FOCUS Technique), breathing becomes better synchronized with the lifting and lowering phase.

Sometimes when I see people exercise in a blatantly careless manner, I ask them if they *really* believe that they're doing what serves them best. I'm still surprised that most reply, "No, I know I'm not!" It surprises me even more when they add, "and I know what I'm doing wrong!" People really do know better, but are afraid to trust their gut. They assume that their instincts are wrong because they're at odds with conventional views.

Top Ten Weight-Training Safety Guidelines

1. *Before using any equipment, check and secure all adjustments.*
2. *Keep your feet, head, and hands away from each machine's moving parts.*
3. *Always maintain a position that is appropriate, strict, and safe.*
4. *Always maintain strict technique (FOCUS).*
5. *Move carefully and methodically from one exercise to another.* Take enough time to make sure all adjustments are properly made and secured.
6. *Use the right tool for the job.* Make sure that whatever you're using is designed for whatever you're doing.
7. *Enlist the help of a spotter when you're working with heavy weights.*
8. *Practice new movements with very light weights before using them in your routine.*
9. *Do not overtrain.* When your muscles are subject to undue stress, there's a greater chance that you'll get hurt.
10. *Always use common sense.* Think about what you plan to do. Ask yourself, before you begin, if it's really worth taking the risk.

Fail to Succeed

Although experts usually agree that we should train to muscular failure, it seems, based on what I've observed, that most people aren't convinced. In fact, a high percentage of folks seem to end each set on a whim. Most perform a random number of vain, "perfunctory" reps.

Unfortunately, when they do this, they don't help themselves at all.

They fail to stress their muscles enough to produce an appreciable change. Instead, they should always try to perform as many strict reps as they can. They should strive, as often as possible, to accomplish muscular failure.

If, when you hear the word "failure," you perceive it as something bad, know that it simply means *don't give up until you're fully fatigued*. Achieving muscular failure means achieving increased success.

Here's an important guideline: If you've been advised to perform in the range of six to ten reps of a movement, select a weight with which you can do at least six before reaching failure. If you're able to do more than ten, then you're not using quite enough weight. The next time you do the same exercise use a heavier weight. If you can't do six repetitions (when using strict FOCUS Technique), you're attempting to use *more* weight than you should and it needs to be *decreased*.

Some experts advise against performing resistance movements to failure. They believe that a lesser effort can accomplish similar gains and provides the added advantage of involving far less risk. Achieving muscular failure, though, involves very little risk—provided a movement is always performed in a slow, strict, and fluid manner. Moreover, my experience is that it's those who do train to failure who improve their bodies faster and to a noticeably greater extent. This isn't to say that it's useless for you to train if you don't work out hard. But your gains are directly related to the intensity of your effort—as long as that effort is always made in a safe and efficient manner.

Others say we should not train to failure more than *one time a week*. They say it's not only unnecessary but also counterproductive. They suggest that a weekly workout plan include a "heavy day" (on which every movement is performed to the point of muscular failure) and a "light day" (training with less weight and a lesser degree of effort). They say that a well-trained muscle needs more time to fully rebuild and that training too hard, too often, is apt to restrict one's rate of success.

Again, my experience is that there's more to gain by training to failure, *unless*: (1) a specific muscle group is trained more than two times a week; (2) you train the same muscle group (maximally) two or more days in succession; (3) more sets are performed than is appropriate; or (4) an exercise is performed wrong. Otherwise, striving for failure is apt to be more productive.

While achieving muscular failure is in many ways beneficial, you should not push yourself in any way that is awkward or uncontrolled. In other words, *stop* if you're using poor form or feeling extreme discomfort. If you haven't been training consistently, or if you haven't been working out long, you need to give your body a chance to adjust to whatever you do. You may also have emotional concerns that affect how you tolerate stress, in which case you must know your limits and be willing to give yourself slack.

Some folks argue that muscular failure can't really be achieved— unless you employ "forced reps" or "eccentric" (lowering) emphasized movements. Although from a technical viewpoint this may in fact be true, unless you're a competitive bodybuilder it's simply not worth the trouble. Not only is it unnecessary, it's also not very practical. For the average person's purposes, a less painful approach will suffice.

Breathing

It's rare that a day goes by that someone fails to ask me this question: What is the best way to breathe when working out with heavy weights? The first thing I usually tell them is, *just make sure that you do*. In other words, whatever you do, don't ever *hold your breath*. Doing so can cause a rise in intrathoracic pressure (the Valsalva maneuver), which can elevate blood pressure markedly when performing resistance movements. This sudden increase in pressure can actually cause you to faint—the last thing you want to have happen while lifting a heavy weight.

When performing any exercise, regardless of your objective, the best advice I can give is to breathe as steadily as you can. Sometimes *exhaling* when *raising* a weight feels more like the right thing to do (this tends to be more often the case when performing pressing movements). Otherwise, what feels most comfortable is likely to serve you best.

Proper breathing helps the mind as much as it does the body. To feel consistently energized and in tune with what you're doing, your breathing must be in harmony with the rhythm of every movement. When your breathing is steady and stable, your energy tends to be too. It's more apt to be consistent and less likely to be short-lived.

Range of Motion

Most experts advise that we lift a weight through a maximum range of motion. Although this is generally good advice, there are some specific exceptions. Certain movements are best performed through only a partial range. The "valueless" part of a movement range is often called the "dead zone." In the dead zone, target muscle groups are not being actively stressed. When lifting a weight through the dead zone, your muscles receive needless rest. Allowing this rest makes a movement much less effective and less intense. Consider performing the free weight squat to understand this point. To perform this movement correctly, these guidelines are often advised: Lower the weight until your thighs are parallel to the floor, then extend the legs to a point that is two-thirds of a full range. When you perform this exercise, full extension is counterproductive, as the last part of the movement (from the two-thirds position to full extension) demands little of the target muscle (quadriceps). Remember, dead zones will vary based on the exercise that you perform. This zone can involve a short or significant part of a movement's full range.

Top Four UFOs with Regard to Performing or Planning Routines

1. INAPPROPRIATE NUMBER OF SETS AND REPETITIONS

Suggested number of sets (for each body part): generally 1–6.
This depends on:

- *Your conditioning level.* For those who are less well-conditioned, less is usually best.
- *Your goals.* You may want to give more attention to particular parts of your body, for example, increasing the strength of your chest, or defining your lower legs.
- *Your exercise technique.* The better your technique is, the better will be your results. With strict technique, you have less need to perform additional sets.

- *Your training intensity*. The greater your training intensity, the less total sets are required.
- *Your strengths and weaknesses*. You may choose to do more for muscle groups that, relatively speaking, are weak.
- *The number of different movements performed for each different part of your body*. The more options you have for each muscle group, the more sets you may choose to perform.

Suggested number of sets, when training different parts of your body

Lower back: 1–2
Neck: 1–2
Trapezius: 1–2
Obliques: 1–2
Inner thigh: 1–2
Outer thigh: 1–2
Forearms: 1–3
Hamstrings: 1–3
Gluteals: 1–3
Abdominals: 1–4
Calves: 1–4
Triceps: 1–4
Biceps: 1–4
Upper back: 1–6
Shoulders: 1–6
Quadriceps: 1–6
Chest: 1–6

*Suggested number of **different movements** for singular body parts*

Fewer than three months of training: no more than 2
Three to six months of training: preferably 2, no more than 3
Six or more months of training: 2–3, no more than 4
Bodybuilder: no more than 4

Repetition ranges

To maximize gains in strength: 3–5
To maximize muscularity: 6–9
For muscle tone *and* endurance: 10–15
For peak muscular endurance: 15+

General responses of muscle groups to ranges of repetitions
Responses are best to lower reps (usually 3–5): traditional, "power" movements such as the dead lift (for the lower back), heavy squats (for the quadriceps and buttocks), and heavy bench presses (for the chest and arms).

Responses are best to medium reps (usually 6–9): chest, upper back, lower back, quadriceps (frontal thigh), hamstrings (posterior thigh), deltoids (shoulders), trapezius, biceps, triceps. *Higher end of range:* calves, forearms, abdominals, neck, and gluteals.

Responses are best to higher reps (usually 10–15): calves, forearms, abdominals, inner thigh (adductors), outer thigh (abductors), gluteals, and obliques.

2. INAPPROPRIATE REST INTERVALS BETWEEN SETS, REPETITIONS, AND WORKOUTS

Suggested rest phase between sets: thirty seconds to two minutes.

Suggested rest phase between repetitions: none. Don't pause—keep consistent tension on the targeted (working) muscles.

Suggested rest phase between workouts: If performing *two* workouts per body part on a regular weekly basis, 72–96 hours between different workouts for the same body part. If performing *three* workouts per body part on a regular weekly basis, 48–72 hours between different workouts for the same body part.

3. INEFFICIENT SEQUENCING OF TRAINING MODES, MOVEMENTS, AND MUSCLE GROUPS

General rules of thumb:

- *Train your larger muscle groups first:* upper back, chest, quadriceps, glutes, hamstrings.
- *Train your smaller muscle groups last:* deltoids, triceps, biceps, forearms, abdominals, calves.
- *When training two large or small muscle groups during a single exercise session, always train those that are tighter, weaker, or less well-developed first.* For example, if during a workout, you're training your chest and your quads (both large muscle groups), always start with the group that is weakest, or lagging behind other groups.
- *Always train the lower back last.* Because most exercises tend to involve your lower back, it shouldn't be heavily stressed or fatigued until you've completed each session. Your lower back must support you while you're performing your other movements.
- *Always train back before biceps.* If you train your biceps first, and work to the point of muscular failure, you won't be able to properly train or isolate your upper back. Your biceps will tire before your upper back can be fully stressed.
- *Always train chest before triceps.* Same rationale as above.
- *Perform all your upper thigh movements before training lower legs.* If you're performing a standing movement, like a lunge or a barbell squat, your position won't be as stable if your calves are already fatigued.
- *Before training inner and outer thighs, perform glute and quadriceps movements.* Same rationale as above.

4. FAILURE TO ADJUST TO PLATEAU PHASES

A plateau phase is a prolonged stretch of time during which progress grinds to a halt. It means that your muscles, essentially, are "bored" with the way you train. To awaken a sluggish body, you must vary the way you work out. Your muscles need some type of stimulus that in some way feels different or new. Here are a few of my favorite ways to shake up a ho-hum routine.

Drop sets

1. Start with the heaviest weight you can use to perform your desired repetitions.
2. Once your muscles are fully fatigued, promptly begin the next set. On the second set, though, reduce the weight, so you're able to do enough reps.

Normally, you'd allow no rest at all between any sets, or just enough rest to strip off weights or to move the pin on a machine. Variations of the drop set technique are performing more than two sets, or resting for various lengths of time between each successive set.

Preexhaustion

1. Select two different movements that mainly target one group of muscles (for example, a press and a lateral raise).
2. Perform a single-joint movement first (for example, the lateral raise).
3. Perform a multijoint movement next (for example, the shoulder press).
4. As soon as you change the weight and/or seat, begin the multijoint movement. Begin this set as fast as you can—don't give yourself any rest.

Single-joint exercises

Biceps curl
Triceps extension
Lateral raise (shoulders)
Dumbbell or "pec deck" fly (chest)
Leg extension (quadriceps)
Leg curl (hamstrings)

Multijoint exercises

Bench press (chest)
Seated press (shoulders)
Squat (quadriceps, buttocks)
Leg press (quadriceps, buttocks)
Close-grip bench press (triceps)
Reverse-grip pulldown (biceps, upper back)
Dips (chest, triceps, shoulders)

Modified Compound Set
1. Select two different movements that will stress different groups of muscles (for example, curls and calf raises).
2. During the time that you normally rest (between sets of the same movement), perform unrelated movements (like the calf raise between sets of curls).

Giant Sets
Perform two or more different movements targeting one muscle group in succession (for example, bench presses, flys, and dips, without any rest in between).

Supersets
1. In succession, perform different movements that target antagonist groups (for example, a triceps extension and then a biceps curl).
2. Always begin the next movement as soon as the first movement is complete. Don't allow any rest between the first and second set.

Examples of superset pairings

Tricep extensions and bicep curls
Leg extensions and leg curls
Pulldowns and seated presses
Bench presses and seated rows
Ab crunches and back extensions
Hip adduction and hip abduction

Weight Training Technique UFOs: Common Problems, Uncommon Solutions

MOVING TOO FAST

Rehearse each exercise mentally before you begin your routine. Imagine all of your movements performed in a slow and fluid fashion. Be more aware of this rhythm and flow whenever you exercise. Develop a pre-workout ritual that helps you to slow your pace (deep, focused breathing, or a sequence of favorite stretches). Try to perform it consistently *before* you begin to work out. Be aware of the things you do whenever you move too fast, like holding your breath, falling off balance, or moving wrong parts of your body. Focus on the word FOCUS— Fluid, Optimally Controlled, Ultra-Slow.

USING EXTRANEOUS MUSCLE GROUPS

Be more conscious of when and where you feel the most stress on your muscles. Consider whether you're using a heavier weight than you really need. Are you shrugging your shoulders, arching your back, or moving wrong parts of your body? Anchor the parts of your body that are most apt to move the wrong way (for example, when you're performing a curl, if your upper arms tend to move, hold or squeeze them tight to your trunk so they don't move forward or back). At first, use machines that enable you to maintain a secure position. Focus on basic movements that are easy to do with strict form.

INCORRECT POSITIONING

Ensure that the pivotal joint is aligned with the center of each machine's cam (often marked with a red dot). Read all directions thoroughly. Always question the accuracy of all equipment adjustments, especially when feeling discomfort or stress on extraneous muscles. Experiment with different positions. Move slowly with a light resistance to see which are most effective.

"FAILING TO FAIL"

Anticipate how many reps you can do and then choose a *higher* number. Next, count each rep *backward*: 20, 19, 18, etc. (This can be disorienting, but in a positive sense—you forget about how many reps you've done or how many more you should do.) You may also want to perform a set without counting reps at all, or perhaps even train with a partner who inspires you to exercise harder.

AWKWARD, LABORED BREATHING; STRAINING AND HOLDING YOUR BREATH

Never tense your neck or face or hold onto bars too tightly. Always use very controlled technique and a weight you can lift with good form. Have a partner remind you to breathe in a stable, consistent manner. If during or after an exercise you consistently feel light-headed, you're probably straining and holding your breath much more than is safe or sound.

POOR KINESTHETIC SENSE

This basically means not knowing how muscles should feel when they're properly stressed. Practice tensing one at a time the muscles you want to target. By doing so, you'll improve your sense of how they should feel when you train. Learn how various movements should stress different parts of your body. If you're failing to stress the right area, you should reassess your technique.

INCONSISTENT MOVEMENT SPEED

Whenever your muscles begin to fatigue, remind yourself of the following: Performing one extra rep *slowly* is better than rushing through several more fast. Keep in mind that you're apt to speed up as an exercise nears completion. Always perform each movement at the same slow rate of speed. For a more objective perspective, you may want to enlist some help. Have someone give you feedback about the consistency of your pace.

ALTERING YOUR TECHNIQUE WHEN FEELING DISCOMFORT OR FATIGUE

Watch yourself in a mirror. If you're rocking, swaying, arching your back, or tensing your neck and shoulders, you're pushing yourself well past the point where you'll realize any gain. Never force a movement by using faulty or reckless technique. It's better to *stop* exercising than to keep doing reps with poor form. The greater the number of body parts you stress when you lift a weight, the more likely it is that you're not working out in a strict and/or stable way.

EXCESSIVE JOINT STRAIN

Always consult your physician before attempting to stress injured joints. Never attempt to use heavy weights (particularly free weights) without using the FOCUS Technique. Until you've increased your strength somewhat and developed a feel for what's right, use machines (instead of free weights) more often throughout your routine. If you're using some type of equipment at home, or using machines at the gym, make sure that all pads, seats, and grips are adjusted correctly to your proportions. Make certain that all range adjustments have been tailored to meet your needs. Wear good, supportive footwear at all times when you train. When appropriate, wrap knees and ankles with an elasticized support (to determine if this would benefit you, consult your medical doctor).

CONSISTENT LACK OF FOCUS, PROBLEMS WITH CONCENTRATION

Focus on the process as opposed to on the result. Practice relaxation techniques to become more in tune with your body. Practice moving your body in a variety of different ways. If you find you have trouble focusing, work out in a more private place (your home or office). Listen to music that motivates you and that helps you to find your "zone." You might want to use a Walkman (as long as you don't try to follow the beat).

DANGEROUS OR INAPPROPRIATE EXERCISE MODIFICATIONS

Don't make a change that in any way: (a) prevents a target muscle group from being thoroughly stressed; (b) decreases intensity; (c) feels awkward or painful; or (d) could cause you injury. Test new techniques with a very light weight before trying a maximum lift.

INAPPROPRIATE RANGE OF MOTION

Whenever you practice an exercise, focus on how it feels. Be mindful of where you feel the greatest amount of "good" muscular stress (good stress is felt in your muscles; bad stress is felt in your joints). Move only through the part of a range where your muscles are feeling "good stress." Avoid exercising in "dead zones," the parts of a range of motion that fail to challenge your target muscles. When using exercise machines, make appropriate range adjustments based on your limitations (if performing the leg extension causes pain when your leg is straight, preset the range adjustment to prevent maximum extension).

LACK OF CONSIDERATION FOR INDIVIDUAL LIMITATIONS

Be honest with yourself about your physical limitations. Remember, what works for someone else may not be right for you. Be more in tune with your body. Consider all of the variables that are critical to your success (skill level, flexibility, coordination, physical status, level of concentration, and sense of balance). If you're limited in these areas, or you've failed to give them much thought, you may have to change or omit some things to accommodate more of your needs.

PERFORMING A LIFT IN A WAY THAT'S UNSAFE OR BIOMECHANICALLY FLAWED

Think isolation. In general, consider the following when assessing your training technique: The more muscles used during an exercise, the less it stimulates growth. Never move parts of your body that you shouldn't or don't have to move (for example, don't arch your back when performing a bench press or biceps curl). If a movement causes discomfort or feels like an awkward thing to do, examine your technique carefully to determine the reason why. Be sure all adjustments are properly made with regard to your body's proportions, as well as with regard to your joint and muscular limitations.

RAISING, SHRUGGING, OR TENSING THE SHOULDERS WHEN TRAINING THE UPPER BODY

When training your upper body in a standing or seated position, face a mirror to see if you're shrugging or tensing your neck or your shoulders. Try not to raise your shoulders at any time during a lift, especially when you're performing: (a) the pulldown, curl, or lateral raise (in a seated or standing position); (b) the cable tricep extension (in the standing or kneeling position); and (c) the chest press, fly, row, or tricep extension (in a seated or inclined position). You may also ask a "spotter" to press down (lightly) on your shoulders. This prevents you from raising them and from using extraneous muscles.

ARCHING THE BACK, ESPECIALLY WHEN PERFORMING PRESSING MOVEMENTS

Avoid all free-standing (nonsupported) free weight pressing movements. Position yourself instead on a seat or a bench that supports your back. Press your lower back *flat* against the bench or back of the seat. Always try to observe your technique by training in front of a mirror. Work with a training partner. Have your partner place his or her hand behind the small of your back. While pressing back on his or her hand, pull in and tighten your abs. This helps you to keep yourself in a stable workout position.

USING MOMENTUM

Practice as much as possible using proper FOCUS Technique. Avoid bouncing, jerking, swinging, flinging, cheating, or forcing a movement. Always keep joints stable and in a strict, consistent position. Pay attention to where you feel the most stress on your muscles. If it's mostly at the start of a lift, you're probably using momentum. Keep belts securely fastened whenever you use machines. Use only a weight that you can lift with flawless FOCUS form.

FAILING TO STABILIZE JOINTS

This is more often a problem when performing a single-joint movement (for example, the biceps curl, tricep extension, leg extension, and leg curl). Always secure your position whenever you use machines. This can be accomplished by: (a) keeping your back against the bench or seat back at all times; (b) when possible, using a seat belt whenever you use machines; and (c) aligning the pivotal joint with the center of each machine's cam. When performing upper arm movements, keep your arms in a fixed position (for example, the back of your upper arms held flush against a wall). You can also anchor your arms by holding them firmly against your sides. Never allow your upper arms to move forward, out, or back. Likewise, if training hamstrings in a supine or standing position, make certain that the front of your leg stays in contact with the machine. Exercise next to a mirror to assess your training technique.

Top Ten Fitness Fallacies

1. *Repetitious, rhythmic exercise is effective for spot reduction.*
2. *The best way to get rid of love handles is to do lots of side bends and twists.*
3. *More is always better.*
4. *When you train with weights, you lose less weight because muscle weighs more than fat.*
5. *No pain, no gain (should be: "no effort, no gain").*
6. *The most effective way to improve your muscular definition is to train with a light resistance while performing numerous reps.*
7. *Some folks are too old to exercise.*
8. *Weight lifting is bad for the heart.*
9. *Sit-ups are the best exercise to banish a sagging gut.*
10. *If you build yourself up and stop working out, your muscles will turn to fat.*

Where Do I Go from Here?

Tailoring Your Program to Meet Your Personal Needs

Be careful about reading health books. You may die of a misprint.

—Mark Twain

Fitness experts often profess, "There's no excuse not to work out. Make exercise a priority—make sure it's first on your list!" Then they suggest that by heeding this trite, oversimplified bit of advice, you're sure to discover that getting in shape isn't nearly as hard as you think. Even the Nike slogan seems to imply that it should be a snap. Whenever I hear "Just do it," I think, "That attitude seems kind of smug." It implies that if people just got off their duffs and stopped coming up with excuses, there wouldn't be anything else in their way to prevent them from reaching their goals. If you haven't figured it out by now, I don't believe this is true. Maybe you can't "just do it?" It's *okay* if you can't just do it! You really do have excuses for why your workouts aren't working out. It's not just about trying harder, being tenacious, or toughening up. It's about overcoming the UFOs that are blocking your path to success.

By now, I hope you've gained insight into your primary UFOs. Perhaps this book has provided you clues about what's *really* been in your way. Let's say it has, and now here you are, wondering what you should do next. Here are some basic guidelines to give you a sense of how to proceed.

How to Develop a Game Plan to Conquer Your UFOs

Take some time to examine the following list of UFOs. For each (based on the following scale) that you rate *between 3 and 5*, write the appropriate number in the space next to each UFO.

UFO RATING SCALE

1: I can't relate at all to the signs and symptoms of this UFO.

2: I can relate a little to signs and symptoms of this UFO.

3: I can somewhat relate to some of the signs and symptoms of this UFO.

4: I relate very much to most of the signs and symptoms of this UFO.

5: I relate to virtually all of the signs and symptoms of this UFO.

SELF-TEST UFOs

—— Psychological reversal (_____)

—— Energy blocks (_____)

—— Appearance obsession

—— Depression, major

—— Depression, low-grade

—— Perfectionism

—— Attention deficit disorder (ADD)

—— Seasonal affective disorder (SAD)

—— Premenstrual syndrome (PMS)

—— Sleep disorders (_____)

—— Subluxations or joint misalignments

—— Chemical, seasonal, or environmental allergies (_____)

—— Medication side-effects (_____)

—— Insulin-sensitivity

—— Food allergies or intolerances (_____)

OTHER UFOs

—— Narrow or shallow perspective (focused on only your body)

—— Self-sabotage (_____)

—— Suppressed emotional conflicts (_____)

—— Overly focused on goals (unable to trust the process)

—— Inner or spiritual void (failing to follow your heart)

—— Lack of self-acceptance

—— Pursuing unhealthy ideals

—— Often derailed by ego-concerns (_____)

—— Distorted perspective of others (buying into a "fitness ideal")

—— Trusting advice that is suspect ("fitness naiveté")

—— Using dangerous drugs

—— Repressed anger and passive-aggression

—— Using your weight as a "wall"

—— Failing to set clear boundaries

—— Exercise addiction

—— Body image or eating disorder (_____)

—— Lack of time

—— Lack of motivation

—— Lack of discipline

—— Hormone imbalance (_____)

—— Not training right for your body type

—— Not training right for your fitness type

—— Genetic limitations (_____)

—— Unhealthy views about diets (_____)

—— Inappropriate balance of protein, fat, and carbs

—— Improper food combining

—— Supplement misconceptions (_____)

—— Improper use of supplements

—— Inefficient food distribution throughout the course of a day

—— Frequent exposure to fattening or unhealthy choices of food (such as

_____)

—— Improper aerobic warm-up

—— Metabolic misconceptions with regard to aerobic intensity

—— Improper use of equipment

—— Failing to vary the training mode

—— Obsession with burning calories

—— Overtraining

—— Undertraining

—— Inconsistent intensity (cardiovascular)

—— Poor timing (working out at inopportune times)

—— Moving too fast when weight training

—— Performing too many reps

—— Ignoring safety considerations (_____)

—— Failing to reach muscle failure

—— Lack of attention to breathing

—— Incorrect range of motion

—— Performing too many sets

—— Inappropriate rest intervals

—— Inefficient sequencing of training modes, movements, and muscle groups

—— Failing to adjust to plateau phases

—— Poor weight-training technique (_____)

—— Other (_____)

Now list your top five UFOs, with your top fitness block listed first. List the remainder in order (putting those with the highest scores first).

Go back through this book and review my advice with regard to your top UFO. Implement all of the steps that you can, and then reassess your status. If your top UFO is no longer a block, it's time to refigure your list. If it still is a block but no longer is first, address what comes *next* on your list.

Continue addressing each UFO until it is under control. Remember, each time you eliminate one, it's important to make a new list. Then, reassess your strategy, based on your new number-one UFO (for example, if restless sleep becomes your primary UFO, it's important to shift your focus with regard to addressing your blocks).

When you do this, you peel back the layers, one by one, to see where you stand. It may be that curbing your top UFO eliminates other blocks too. More often, though, it helps "clear the brush," so you see what remains in your way. By going at this methodically, you catch things you'd otherwise miss. Your perspective of what's really holding you back will be clearer to you every day.

While in the throes of writing this book, I received a great deal of advice. But it's what a good friend of mine said to me once that I recollect most of all.

"Here's what you gotta do," he said. "Trust me, I know these things. Come up with some sort of radical plan that's never before been revealed. Tell people you've found this great new way to get into shape really fast, without any struggle or effort at all and without any ill effects. Promise them something, anything, as long as it's different or new."

"I'm not quite sure what you mean," I replied. "What do you think I should say?"

"It doesn't matter," he said with a laugh. "Tell them whatever you want. Tell them that to lose cellulite, a belt sander works like a charm, or that new studies show Velveeta cheese is an excellent fat-burning food! Tell people something radical, and your message will be a big hit."

"I do have a radical message," I said. "It's all about moving past blocks. It's all about finding the missing links to getting, and staying, in shape."

"Stop being such an idealist," he said. "Remember, you want to sell books! Besides, most people can't handle the truth—it's too hard for them to accept. Promise them something outrageous, even if you have to lie!"

"I'd rather be an idealist," I said, "than tell people some kind of lie. People are starting to realize now that there isn't one path to success. They're longing to hear a message that, for once, isn't trite or contrived. They've had it with experts who don't walk their talk, or who can't comprehend how they feel. They're ready to hear a new message, one that accounts for their own, unique needs."

I hope it turns out that I'm right about this, and I'm not simply being naive. I firmly believe that people are tired of looking for some magic pill. They're starting to see that it doesn't exist, that there's no secret way to get fit. People are wising up to the fact that they must follow different paths. They're tired of jumping on bandwagons. They're tired of falling off!

Here is my humble prediction—you can say that you read it here first. After the turn of the century, our perspectives on fitness will change. We'll see that the things we obsess about now are the things that restrict our success. We'll be less obsessed about image concerns and more called to connect with our soul. We'll learn how to play with the hand we've been dealt and to win at our *own* fitness game.

Appendix

Chapter 1

RESOURCES

Thought-Field Therapy

Roger Callahan, Ph.D.
The Callahan Techniques
45-350 Vista Santa Rosa
Indian Wells, CA 92210
(619) 345-9216
(800) 359-CURE
Fax: (619) 360-5258
Web site: http://www.tftrx.com

Finding a Certified Therapist

National Board for Certified Counselors
(336) 547-0607 (Monday-Friday, 8:30 A.M.-4:30 P.M., Eastern time)
E-mail: nbcc@nbcc.org. Include your name, mailing address, location where
you're seeking a counselor, and type of counselor you're seeking. Lists cannot be E-mailed.

National Mental Health Association (NMHA)
(800) 969-NMHA

American Psychiatric Association
(202) 682-6800
to locate a psychiatrist or psychopharmacologist

American Psychological Association
(202) 336-5700
to locate a clinical psychologist

American Counseling Association
(703) 823-9800
to locate a professional counselor

American Association for Marriage and Family Therapy
(202) 452-0109
to locate a marriage and family therapist

National Association of Social Workers
(800) 683-9799
to locate a clinical social worker

BOOKS
Mind-Body

Your Body Believes Every Word You Say by Barbara Hoberman Levine (Lower Lake, CA: Aslan Publishing, 1991)

Psychological Kinesiology: Changing the Body's Beliefs by William F. Whisenant (Kailua, HI: Monarch Butterfly Productions, 1994)

Thought-Field Therapy

Why Do I Eat When I'm Not Hungry? How to Use Your Body's Own Energy System to Treat Food Addictions by Roger Callahan, Ph.D. (New York: Doubleday, 1991)

Journaling

Journal to the Soul: The Art of Sacred Journal Keeping by Rose Offner (Layton, UT: Gibbs-Smith, 1996)

General Health

8 Weeks to Optimum Health by Andrew Weil, M.D. (New York: Alfred A. Knopf, 1997)

The Future of the Body: Explorations Into the Further Evolution of Human Nature by Michael Murphy (Los Angeles: Jeremy Tarcher, 1992)

Ageless Body, Timeless Mind by Deepak Chopra, M.D. (New York: Harmony Books, 1993)

NEWSLETTER

Dr. Andrew Weil's *Self-Healing* newsletter
To order: (800) 523-3926
12 issues for $29

Chapter 2

BOOKS

Inspiration

Awakening the Buddha Within: Eight Steps to Enlightenment—Tibetan Wisdom for the Western World by Lama Surya Das (New York: Broadway Books, 1998)

The Book of Practical Faith by D. Patrick Miller (New York: Henry Holt, 1995)

Spiritual Healing

Anatomy of the Spirit: The Seven Steps of Power and Healing by Caroline Myss, Ph.D. (New York: Harmony Books, 1996)

Connecting With Your Heart

The Artist's Way: A Spiritual Path to Higher Creativity by Julia Cameron (Los Angeles: Jeremy Tarcher, 1992)

Chapter 3

BOOKS

Appearance Obsession

Appearance Obsession: Learning to Love the Way You Look by Joni E. Johnston, Psy.D. (Deerfield Beach, FL: Health Communications, 1994)

The Beauty Myth by Naomi Wolf (New York: Doubleday, 1991)

Love the Body You Were Born With: A Ten Step Workbook for Women by Monica Dixon (New York: Perigee, 1994)

Real Gorgeous: The Truth About Body and Beauty by Kaz Cooke (New York: Norton, 1996)

Exercise Addiction

Hooked On Exercise: How to Understand and Manage Exercise Addiction by Rebecca Prussin, M.D., Philip Harvey, Ph.D., and Theresa Foy DiGeronimo (New York: Simon & Schuster, 1992)

Steroids/Performance-Enhancement Drugs

Muscle: Confessions of an Unlikely Bodybuilder by Samuel Wilson Fussell (New York: Avon Books, 1991)

ASSOCIATION

National Council on Alcoholism and Drug Dependence
12 West 21 Street, 8th Floor
New York, NY 10010
(800) 423-4673
(212) 206-6770

RESOURCE

Professional Image Consultant

Ginger Burr
Total Image Consultants
15 Fenwick Street, #2
Somerville, MA 02145
(617) 665-5225

Chapter 4

BOOKS

Imago Relationship Therapy

Keeping the Love You Find by Harville Hendrix, Ph.D. (New York: Pocket Books, 1992)

Depression

Living With Prozac: Personal Accounts of Life on Anti-Depressants by Debra Elfenbein, ed. (New York: Scribner, 1997)

Nutrition and Mental Illness: An Orthomolecular Approach to Balancing Body Chemistry by Carl C. Pfeiffer (Rochester, VT: Healing Arts Press, 1987)

Dealing With Depression Naturally: The Drugless Approach to the Condition That Darkens Millions of Lives by Syd Baumel (New Canaan, CT: Keats Publishing, 1995)

I Don't Want to Talk About It: Overcoming the Secret Legacy of Male Depression by Terrence Real (New York: Scribner, 1997)

You Mean, I Don't Have to Feel This Way? New Help For Depression, Anxiety, and Addiction by Colette Dowling (New York: Scribner, 1991)

Perfectionism

Too Perfect—When Being in Control Gets Out of Control by Allan E. Mallinger, M.D., and Jeannette DeWyze (New York: Clarkson Potter, 1992)

Body Image/Eating Disorders

Thin Disguise: Understanding and Overcoming Anorexia and Bulimia by Pam Vredevelt, Deborah Newman, Harry Beverly, and Frank Minirth (Nashville, TN: Nelson, 1992)

Hunger Pains—From Fad Diets to Eating Disorders: What Every Woman Needs to Know About Food, Dieting, and Self-Concept by Mary Pipher (Holbrook, MA: Adams Publishing, 1995)

Stop Being Mean to Yourself by Melody Beattie (San Francisco: HarperCollins, 1997)

Breaking Free From Compulsive Eating by Geneen Roth (New York: Signet, 1984)

Feeding the Hungry Heart: The Experience of Compulsive Eating by Geneen Roth (New York: Signet, 1982)

Daring to Be Yourself by Alexandra Stoddard (New York: Doubleday, 1991)

Lack of Time, Motivation, and Discipline

Take Time for Your Life: A Personal Coach's 7 Step Program for Creating the Life You Want by Cheryl Richardson (New York: Broadway Books, 1998)

Too Busy to Exercise by Porter Shimer (Pownal, VT: Storey Communications, 1996)

Fitting in Fitness: Hundreds of Simple Ways to Put More Physical Activity Into Your Life by the American Heart Association (New York: Times Books, 1997)

Getting Unstuck: Breaking Through Your Barriers to Change by Sidney B. Simon (New York: Warner Books, 1989)

PRODUCT INFORMATION

Electroacupuncture

Healthpoint
To order: Dove Marketing, Ltd.
      3A Ashley Road, Altrincham
      Cheshire, WA14 2DN, England
      U.S. Hotline: (800) 455-9155

RESOURCE

Imago Relationship Coach

Edward Shea
239 East Wilson
Elmhurst, IL 60126
(630) 530-1060
E-mail: Coachimago@aol.com

Chapter 5

BOOKS

Attention Deficit Disorder

Driven to Distraction by Edward M. Hallowell and John J. Ratey (New York: Pantheon, 1994)

Answers to Distraction by Edward M. Hallowell and John J. Ratey (New York: Pantheon, 1994)

Total Concentration: How to Understand Attention Deficit Disorders by Harold N. Levinson (New York: M. Evans, 1992)

Out of the Fog: Treatment Options and Coping Strategies for Adult ADD by Kevin R. Murphy and Suzanne LeVert (New York: Hyperion, 1995)

Premenstrual Syndrome

Women's Bodies, Women's Wisdom: Creating Physical and Emotional Health and Healing by Christiane Northrup, M.D. (New York: Bantam Books, 1998)

Acupressure

Acupressure's Potent Points: A Guide to Self-Care for Common Ailments by Michael Reed Gach (New York: Bantam Books, 1990)

Seasonal Affective Disorder

Seasons of the Mind: Why You Get the Winter Blues & What You Can Do About It by Norman E. Rosenthal, M.D. (New York: Guilford Press, 1993)

Fight the Winter Blues—Don't Be Sad: Your Guide to Conquering Seasonal Affective Disorder by Celeste A. Peters (Calgary, Alberta Canada: Script Publishing, 1994)

Sleep Disorders

Sleep Thieves: An Eye-Opening Exploration Into the Science and Mysteries of Sleep by Stanley Coren (New York: Free Press, 1996)

*Power Sleep: The Revolutionary Program That Prepares Your Mind for Peak
Performance* by Dr. James B. Maas (New York: Villard, 1998)

Hormone Imbalances
The SuperHormone Promise: Nature's Antidote to Aging by William Regelson, M.D., and Carol Colman (New York: Pocket Books, 1996)

PRODUCT INFORMATION
Bright Light Sources

The SunBox Company
19217 Orbit Drive
Gaithersburg, MD 20879
(800) LITE-YOU
(800) 548-3968
(301) 869-5980

Apollo Light Systems, Inc.
352 West 1060 South
Orem, UT 84058
(800) 545-9667
(801) 226-2370

Medic-Light, Inc.
Yacht Club Drive
Lake Hopatcong, NJ 07849
(800) LIGHT-25
(201) 663-1214

NEWSLETTER

Dr. Christiane Northrup's *Health Wisdom For Women* newsletter
Phillips Publishing, Inc.
7811 Montrose Road
Potomac, MD 20854
(800) 804-0935
12 issues for $39.95

FOR ADDITIONAL INFORMATION

Society for Light Treatment and Biological Rhythms
Francine Butler, Executive Director
West 44th Avenue
Suite 304-10200
Wheat Ridge, CO 80033
(303) 424-3697

For a fee of $7, this organization will provide an SAD information packet that includes questions and answers about bright light therapy, bibliographies of recent works in the field, a list of research centers, and a geographically appropriate list of SLTBR members who are accepting patient inquiries. Send a self-addressed, stamped envelope (along with your check) or order directly from the Web site (http://www.websciences.org/sltbr/>).

To locate a support group:
NOSAD
PO Box 40133
Washington, DC 20016

ADD Coaches
National Coaching Network
Box 353
Lafayette Hill, PA 19444
For information, send $3 and a self-addressed, stamped business envelope.

ADD Organizations
Attention Deficit Disorder Association (ADDA)
PO Box 488
West Newbury, MA 01985

Adult ADD Association
1225 East Sunset Drive
Suite 640
Bellingham, WA 98226-3529
(206) 647-6681

ADD Newsletter
ADDendum
C/O C.P.S.
5041-A Backlick Road
Annandale, VA 22003
For adults with ADD, lists adult ADD support groups.

Thyroid Disorders
Thyroid Foundation of America
(800) 832-8231
Web site: www.tfaweb.org/pub/tfa

Chapter 6

BOOKS

Environmental Allergies
Cross Currents: The Perils of Electropollution/The Promise of Electrome-dicine by Robert O. Becker (Los Angeles: Jeremy Tarcher, 1990)

Ayurvedic Body Types
Body, Mind, and Sport: The Mind-Body Guide to Lifelong Fitness and Your Personal Best by John Douillard (New York: Harmony Books, 1994)

Chapter 7

BOOKS

Insulin-Sensitivity
Enter the Zone by Barry Sears, Ph.D. (New York: HarperCollins, 1995)
Mastering the Zone: The Next Step in Achieving SuperHealth and Permanent Fat Loss by Barry Sears, Ph.D. (New York: HarperCollins, 1997)
The Carbohydrate Addict's Diet: The Lifelong Solution to Yo-Yo Dieting by Dr. Rachael F. Heller and Dr. Richard F. Heller (New York: Signet, 1993)

Cravings
Why Do I Eat When I'm Not Hungry? How to Use Your Body's Own Energy System to Treat Food Addictions by Roger Callahan, Ph.D. (New York: Doubleday, 1991)
Overcoming Overeating by Jane Hirschmann and Carol M. Munter (New York: Fawcett Columbine, 1989)

Food Combining

Fit for Life 2 by Harvey and Marilyn Diamond (New York: Warner Books, 1987)

Supplementation

Healthy Healing: An Alternative Healing Reference by Linda G. Rector-Page, N.D., Ph.D. (Carmel Valley, CA: Healthy Healing Publications, 1992)

A Prescription for Nutritional Healing—A Practical A-Z Reference to Drug-Free Remedies Using Vitamins, Minerals, Herbs, and Food Supplements by James F. Balch, M.D., and Phyllis A. Balch, C.N.C. (Garden City Park, NY: Avery Publishing, 1990)

Are You Confused? by Dr. Paavo Airola (Sherwood, OR: Health Plus, 1995)

Creatine: Nature's Muscle Builder by Ray Sahelian, M.D., and Dave Tuttle (Garden City Park, NY: Avery Publishing Group, 1997)

Other

The Balance: Your Personal Prescription for Supermetabolism, Renewed Vitality, Maximum Health, and Instant Rejuvenation by Oz Garcia (New York: HarperCollins, 1998)

SUPPLEMENTS WORTH LOOKING INTO

Barleygreen
AIM International
3904 E. Flamingo Avenue
Nampa, ID 83687-3100
(800) 456-2462

PureSynergy Superfood
The Synergy Company
CVSR Box 2901
Moab, UT 84532
(800) 723-0277
Web site: http://www.synergy-co.com

RESOURCES

Nutritional Intuitive/Dietitian

Halé Baycu-Schatz
PO Box 504
Lexington, MA 02173
(781) 863-9997

Energy Healer, Addiction Specialist, and Medical/Nutritional Intuitive
Rhonda Lenair
The Lenair Technique, Inc.
75 Scotland Road
Newbury, MA 01951
(978) 465-7711

Biodermal Assay/Individualized Supplement Prescription
Kenneth Emonds, Ph.D.
New England Center for Environmental Medicine
65 Newburyport Turnpike
Newbury, MA 01951
(978) 465-5009

PRODUCT INFORMATION

Diet Coach (Electronic Organizer)
Diet Coach
To order: (800) 346-4637 (9 A.M. to 5 P.M. Central time)

Handheld Diet and Nutrition Guide (Electronic Organizer)
Inner Balance
360 Interlocken Boulevard, Suite 300
Broomfield, CO 80021
To order: (800) 482-3608
Fax: (800) 456-1139

Chapter 8

BOOKS

General Fitness
Health & Fitness Excellence: The Comprehensive Action Plan by Robert K. Cooper (Boston: Houghton Mifflin, 1989)
Fitness for Dummies by Suzanne Scholsberg and Liz Neporent (San Mateo, CA: IDG Books, 1996)

Aerobics/Cardiovascular
Smart Exercise: Burning Fat, Getting Fit by Covert Bailey (Boston: Houghton Mifflin, 1994)
The Aerobics Program for Total Well-Being by Dr. Kenneth H. Cooper (New York: M. Evans, 1982)

Chapter 9

BOOKS

Strength Fitness: Physiological Principles and Training Techniques by Wayne Wescott, Ph.D. (Dubuque, IA: Wm. C. Brown, 1995)

Kinesiology of Exercise by Michael Yessis, Ph.D. (Indianapolis: Masters Press, 1992)

A Practical Approach to Strength Training by Matt Brzycki (Indianapolis: Masters Press, 1991)

Weight Training: Steps to Success by Thomas R. Baechle and Barney R. Groves (Champaign, IL: Leisure Press, 1992)

Index

ABOUT THE AUTHOR

Michael Gerrish, M.S., is an exercise physiologist, counseling psycho-therapist, certified thought-field therapist, and former Ford (Boston) model. He was a conditioning consultant for the Boston Red Sox and Boston Bruins, and he is considered one of the country's top holistic fitness professionals. He lives in Massachusetts.

To contact the author:

Michael Gerrish
PO Box 13
Newburyport, MA 01950
E-mail: michael@michaelgerrish.com